Informing the Future
Critical Issues in Health

FIFTH EDITION

INSTITUTE OF MEDICINE
OF THE NATIONAL ACADEMIES

INSTITUTE OF MEDICINE   **500 Fifth Street, N.W.**   **Washington, DC 20001**

Funding: This document was produced using internal IOM funds.

The **National Academy of Sciences** is a private, nonprofit, self-perpetuating society of distinguished scholars engaged in scientific and engineering research, dedicated to the furtherance of science and technology and to their use for the general welfare. Upon the authority of the charter granted to it by the Congress in 1863, the Academy has a mandate that requires it to advise the federal government on scientific and technical matters. Dr. Ralph J. Cicerone is president of the National Academy of Sciences.

The **National Academy of Engineering** was established in 1964, under the charter of the National Academy of Sciences, as a parallel organization of outstanding engineers. It is autonomous in its administration and in the selection of its members, sharing with the National Academy of Sciences the responsibility for advising the federal government. The National Academy of Engineering also sponsors engineering programs aimed at meeting national needs, encourages education and research, and recognizes the superior achievements of engineers. Dr. Charles M. Vest is president of the National Academy of Engineering.

The **Institute of Medicine** was established in 1970 by the National Academy of Sciences to secure the services of eminent members of appropriate professions in the examination of policy matters pertaining to the health of the public. The Institute acts under the responsibility given to the National Academy of Sciences by its congressional charter to be an adviser to the federal government and, upon its own initiative, to identify issues of medical care, research, and education. Dr. Harvey V. Fineberg is president of the Institute of Medicine.

The **National Research Council** was organized by the National Academy of Sciences in 1916 to associate the broad community of science and technology with the Academy's purposes of furthering knowledge and advising the federal government. Functioning in accordance with general policies determined by the Academy, the Council has become the principal operating agency of both the National Academy of Sciences and the National Academy of Engineering in providing services to the government, the public, and the scientific and engineering communities. The Council is administered jointly by both Academies and the Institute of Medicine. Dr. Ralph J. Cicerone and Dr. Charles M. Vest are chair and vice chair, respectively, of the National Research Council.

For more information about the Institute of Medicine, visit the IOM home page at: **www.iom.edu**.

Copyright 2009 by the National Academy of Sciences. All rights reserved.

Printed in the United States of America

The serpent has been a symbol of long life, healing, and knowledge among almost all cultures and religions since the beginning of recorded history. The serpent adopted as a logotype by the Institute of Medicine is a relief carving from ancient Greece, now held by the Staatliche Museen in Berlin.

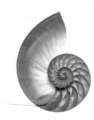

COVER: The nautilus shell is a marvel of the natural world. As the nautilus matures, its shell expands geometrically to accommodate the growing shell-fish, unfolding into a functional home as well as one of nature's perfect logarithmic spirals. First expressed by Descartes, the logarithmic spiral underlies not only the nautilus shell but also much of the natural world, including the human cochlea, the Milky Way, and a simple pinecone.

Suggested citation: IOM (Institute of Medicine). 2009. *Informing the Future: Critical Issues in Health, Fifth Edition.* Washington, DC: The National Academies Press.

"Knowing is not enough; we must apply.
Willing is not enough; we must do."
—Goethe

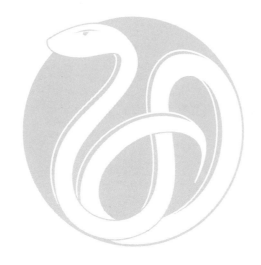

INSTITUTE OF MEDICINE
OF THE NATIONAL ACADEMIES

Advising the Nation. Improving Health.

Contents

The Institute of Medicine: Advising the Nation, Improving Health

The Institute of Medicine (IOM) is an independent, nonprofit organization that works outside of government to provide unbiased and authoritative advice to decision makers and the public. Established in 1970, the IOM is the health arm of the National Academy of Sciences, which was chartered under President Abraham Lincoln in 1863.

Nearly 150 years later, the National Academy of Sciences has expanded into what is collectively known as The National Academies, which comprises the National Academy of Sciences, the National Academy of Engineering, the National Research Council, and the IOM.

During the century-and-a-half that has passed, much has changed in the world, particularly in the field of health and medicine. In 1863, for example, doctors conducted surgery, but infection and death were widespread, largely because hands and instruments often went unwashed before surgery. Surgical antisepsis did not begin to spread widely in practice until after the late 1860s. Since then, we have seen the development of vaccines for diseases ranging from tetanus to polio. The world has witnessed the eradication of smallpox, a disease that sickened an estimated 50 million people per year as recently as the early 1950s. During the same time that such major advances were made, new diseases continued to emerge. HIV/AIDS, identified in the early 1980s, has killed millions around the globe. Humans are living longer, more productive lives, but increasing numbers are also burdened by chronic disease. While hunger remains a

1

serious problem in disadvantaged populations, affluent countries such as the United States are experiencing an alarming rise in obesity.

The IOM is well equipped to adapt to such an ever-changing environment.

With a mission to advise the nation on matters of health and medicine, the IOM takes its role very seriously. Many of the studies that the IOM undertakes begin as specific mandates by Congress; still others are requested by federal agencies and independent organizations.

The IOM applies a distinct research process to provide objective and straightforward answers to difficult questions of national importance. Committees who conduct these studies are carefully composed to ensure the requisite expertise and to avoid conflict of interest. These leading national and international scientists, all of whom serve as volunteers, are asked to set aside preconceptions and to rely on evidence in the pursuit of knowledge and truth.

Even after this work is accomplished, the rigorous IOM process is not yet complete. Before any IOM report is released, it undergoes extensive peer review by a second group of experts, which remains anonymous to the authoring committee until the study is published. For nearly 40 years, this process has resulted in sound IOM reports providing policy makers, the health professions, and the American people with objective advice grounded in evidence.

Each year, more than 2,000 individuals, members, and nonmembers volunteer their time, knowledge, and expertise to advance the nation's health through the work of the IOM. Membership in the IOM is offered to 65 individuals each year, elected by the current membership, and drawn from a range of health care professions; the natural, social, and behavioral sciences; and fields such as law, economics, engineering, and the humanities. For those at the top of their field, membership in the Institute of Medicine reflects the height of professional achievement and commitment to service.

The IOM works to improve health through shared knowledge. While expert, consensus committees are vital to its advisory role, the IOM also convenes a series of forums, roundtables, and standing committees to facilitate discussion, discovery, and critical, cross-disciplinary thinking. The forums and roundtables at the IOM bring together leaders in government and industry, scientists and other experts from academia, practitioners, representatives of public interest groups, and consumers. The IOM offers a mutual venue for open dialogue, on topics as complex and diverse as new drug discovery and development, public health and medical preparedness, evidence-based medicine, environmental health sciences, neuroscience and nervous system disorders, health disparities, and microbial threats. At the IOM, individuals of goodwill from diverse perspectives can gain shared understanding and fresh insights. If a topic matters in an important way to health, sooner or later it will find a place on the agenda of the IOM.

In addition, the IOM is home to several fellowship programs. For more than three decades, the IOM has managed The Robert Wood Johnson Foundation Health Policy Fellowships Program, which is designed to develop the capacity of outstanding mid-career health professionals in academic and community-based settings to assume leadership roles in health policy and management.

The body of this book illustrates the work of IOM committees in selected, major areas in recent years, followed by a description of IOM's convening and collaborative activities and fellowship programs. The last section provides a comprehensive bibliography of IOM reports published since 2007.

Charting a Course for the Future of Health Care

Today, perhaps more than ever, health care is a key item on the nation's agenda. Government policy makers, health professionals, scientists, industrial and civic leaders, patient advocates, and private citizens across the social spectrum are focusing on how best to obtain a high-quality health system that is efficient and affordable in its operation and that functions well for everyone.

The Institute of Medicine (IOM) regularly considers this challenge from a variety of perspectives. Recent efforts have focused on improving the organization and operation of the nation's largest health agency; working to assess what diagnostic, therapeutic, and preventive services work best; gauging the overall health of the nation's population; and identifying ways to build an even stronger foundation of evidence-based medicine that effectively captures the promise of scientific discovery and technological innovation and enables doctors, nurses, and other health professionals to provide the right care for the right patient at the right time.

Revitalizing Health and Human Services

The U.S. Department of Health and Human Services (HHS)—the largest of all federal departments, spending approximately $2 billion a day—profoundly affects the lives of all Americans. Its agencies and programs protect against domestic and global health threats, monitor the safety of food and drugs, advance the science of treating and preventing disease, safeguard society's most vulnerable populations, and work to improve health for everyone. However, HHS increasingly faces serious and complex obstacles, chief among them rising health care costs and a broadening range of health challenges. The department also faces internal challenges.

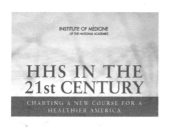
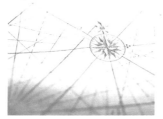

Over time, the federal government has charged HHS with additional responsibilities and removed others, often without corresponding shifts in organizational procedures, structures, or resources.

Recognizing such concerns, Congress asked the IOM to examine whether HHS is "ideally organized" to meet the nation's enduring and emerging health challenges. The study committee's report, *HHS in the 21st Century: Charting a New Course for a Healthier America* (2008), identifies many factors that reduce the department's ability to meet its range of responsibilities. These factors include divergence in the missions and goals of the department's agencies, limited flexibility in spending, impending workforce shortages, difficulty in retaining skilled professionals, and problems in effectively partnering with the private sector.

The report emphasizes the need for HHS to improve performance and processes for goal setting, decision making, management, and accountability—but it does not call for a large-scale reorganization of the entire department. Instead, it seeks action in five specific areas.

Defining a 21st-century vision

HHS currently lacks a clear vision of how to provide the greatest value in protecting and improving health in today's climate of varied, complex, and sometimes changing health needs. By defining such a vision—along with a complementary mission statement that defines a small number of measurable, time-specific goals—HHS can help individuals in Congress, throughout the federal government and the health sector, and across the nation at large to understand the role and importance of the department's work.

HHS—the largest of all federal departments, spending approximately $2 billion a day—profoundly affects the lives of all Americans.

Fostering adaptability and alignment

To best position itself to respond to the nation's health challenges and to adapt quickly to changing circumstances, HHS must align all of its operations more effectively. Furthermore, the leaders of all of its various units should strive to ensure that their activities mesh with the department's overall vision, mission, and goals. Among particular recommendations, HHS should reduce its number of senior-level officials; develop a more prominent and powerful role for the surgeon general; and provide predictable funding for its science agencies, including specific funding for the Agency for Healthcare Research and Quality that is independent of other departmental appropriations.

One area of public health that is ripe for change is food safety, which cannot be addressed adequately within HHS's current structure. The department's food-related agencies are insufficiently equipped and understaffed to keep pace with food safety issues, especially in light of the globalization of the food supply. As an important step, Congress should unify the Department of Agriculture's Food Safety and Inspection Service and the Food and Drug Administration's food safety activities, place the resulting entity under HHS, and provide it with adequate resources for high-quality inspection, enforcement, and research.

Increasing effectiveness and efficiency of the health care system

By all accounts, the nation's current health care system is flawed, marked by rising costs, lack of evidence about the effectiveness of even the most widespread medical procedures, and a growing number of people who are uninsured. Among suggested changes, HHS should work with Congress to establish a capability for assessing the comparative value—including clinical and cost effectiveness—of medical interventions and procedures, preventive and treatment technologies, and methods of organizing and delivering care. This effort will require expanded information sharing, both within the department as well as with external organizations, in order to better evaluate and inform the health care system.

Strengthening the health care workforce

Analysts predict serious shortages across the health care spectrum of people with the right backgrounds, training, and skills. Such shortages will affect not only HHS, but also state and local public health agencies, the private

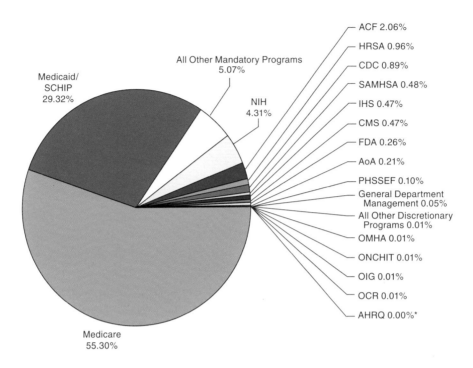

Distribution of HHS actual expenditures, FY 2007.

*The AHRQ is shown as representing 0 percent of the department's budget because it receives funds only from other Public Health Service (PHS) agencies through the PHS evaluation set-aside and has not had its own separate budget allocation since 2002. In fact, the President's budget request for AHRQ has been zero since 2001. Its 2009 program-level expenses were projected at $326 million, making it by far the smallest PHS agency.

NOTE: ACF = Administration for Children and Families; AHRQ = Agency for Healthcare Research and Quality; AoA = Administration on Aging; CDC = Centers for Disease Control and Prevention; CMS = Centers for Medicare and Medicaid Services; FDA = Food and Drug Administration; HRSA = Health Resources and Services Administration; IHS = Indian Health Service; OCR = Office for Civil Rights; OIG = Office of the Inspector General; OMHA = Office of Medicare Hearings and Appeals; ONCHIT = Office of the National Coordinator for Health Information Technology; PHSSEF = Public Health and Social Services Emergency Fund; SAMHSA = Substance Abuse and Mental Health Services Administration; SCHIP = State Children's Health Program, a component of Medicaid.

SOURCE: HHS in the 21st Century: Charting a New Course for a Healthier America, p. 28.

health care sector, and the science establishment. Current workforce challenges include an aging workforce, new health challenges that require new skills, an imbalance between primary care physicians and specialists, and an underrepresentation of minority groups among the nation's health professionals. In this light, HHS should place a high priority on developing a strategy for workforce recruitment and improvement within its own ranks, as well as in the public health and health care professions nationwide, and in the biosciences. Special emphasis should be placed on assessing and addressing the current and projected gaps in the number, professional mix, geographic distribution, and diversity of the nation's public health and health care workforces.

Improving accountability and decision making

A strong system of accountability will provide HHS with the incentive, as well as the information it needs, to improve its performance. Toward this end, Congress and HHS should form a "new compact" that would grant the department greater flexibility in its internal operations and decision making while requiring it to assume greater accountability for assessing its operations. As part of this arrangement, HHS would be required to provide Congress and the public with regular, rigorous reports detailing the department's progress in improving the nation's health.

Although improving the organization and efficiency of HHS will move the nation forward in meeting its health needs, this step alone will not solve the health care crisis. There are many other factors at play, and one critical question is whether doctors are delivering the best care possible. The IOM recently considered this question from multiple perspectives.

Assessing what works in health care

Solving some of the nation's most pressing health policy problems may hinge on the capacity to identify which diagnostic, therapeutic, and preventive services work best for various patients and under various circumstances. As many studies have documented, spending on ineffective care contributes to rising health costs and insurance premiums. Variations in how multiple health care providers treat the same conditions reflect uncertainty and disagreement about what the clinical practice standards should be. Patients and insurers cannot always be confident that health professionals are delivering the best, most effective care. At the same time, health plans are burdened with the need to constantly learn how their covered populations might benefit from—or be harmed by—newly available health services. Meanwhile, some observers argue that consumers who are

> Solving some of the nation's most pressing health policy problems may hinge on the capacity to identify which diagnostic, therapeutic, and preventive services work best for various patients and under various circumstances.

equipped with good information will have the power to reduce the cost and improve the quality of care they receive. Yet even the most sophisticated and motivated health care consumer struggles to learn which care is appropriate for his or her circumstance.

To help correct this problem, The Robert Wood Johnson Foundation asked the IOM to recommend a sustainable, replicable approach to

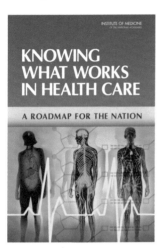

identifying effective clinical services. The resulting report, *Knowing What Works in Health Care: A Roadmap for the Nation* (2008), lays out a detailed action plan. As a key step, Congress should direct HHS to establish a single national program—either a public or joint public–private entity—with the authority, expertise, and resources necessary to set priorities for evaluating clinical services and to conduct systematic reviews of the evidence on clinical effectiveness.

The program should be guided, in part, by an independent advisory committee that would identify high-priority topics that merit systematic evidence assessment. The committee's priority-setting process should be scientifically rigorous, transparent, efficient, and understandable by outsiders. The committee should consider a range of topics, including new, emerging, and well-established health services and technologies for prevention, diagnosis, and treatment. The highest priorities should be the clinical questions of patients and clinicians that have the potential for substantial impact on health outcomes across all ages by reducing the burden of disease, health disparities, and undesirable variation in the delivery of health services

As part of its charge, the program also would develop and promote rigorous standards for creating clinical practice guidelines, which could help clinicians and patients make informed decisions about appropriate health care for specific clinical circumstances, minimize use of questionable services, and target services to the patients most likely to benefit. At present, there are few protections against the proliferation of poorly developed guidelines. Moreover, there is a plethora of guidelines for some conditions (for example, as of 2007 there were more than 471 guidelines just for managing hypertension), and the guidelines sometimes offer conflicting and confusing advice. Guidelines would best be developed by a panel of experts who have access to the fullest array of evidence on a given medical

---

Research Studies

Examples:
* Randomized clinical trials
* Cohort studies
* Case control studies
* Cross-sectional studies
* Case series

↓

Systematic Review
* Identify and assess the quality of individual studies
* Critically appraise the body of evidence
* Develop qualitative or quantitative synthesis

- - - - - - - - - - - - -

↓

Clinical Guidelines and Recommendations

Continuum from research studies to systematic review to development of clinical guidelines and recommendations.

NOTE: The dashed line is the theoretical dividing line between the systematic review of the research literature and its application to clinical decision making, including the development of clinical guidelines and recommendations. Below the dashed line, decision makers and developers of clinical recommendations interpret the findings of systematic reviews to decide which patients, health care settings, or other circumstances they relate to.

SOURCE: Knowing What Works in Health Care: A Roadmap for the Nation, p. 23.

intervention, an understanding of the clinical problem and the appropriate research methods, and sufficient time and resources to absorb the information and make considered judgments.

In response to the report, the federal government has initiated several actions. In June 2008, Congress enacted the Medicare Improvement for Patients and Providers Act, authorizing, among other things, $3 million for IOM studies on recommended standards for conducting systematic reviews and developing clinical practice guidelines. In addition, in July 2008, Senators Kent Conrad (D-ND) and Max Baucus (D-MT) introduced the Comparative Effectiveness Research Act, which incorporates a number of the IOM's recommendations. It calls for a nonprofit entity called the Health Care Comparative Effectiveness Research Institute to set a national research agenda and to "conduct comparative effectiveness research on health interventions." The legislation also would allow the IOM to serve in a consulting role to this institute.

Advancing evidence-based health care

American medicine has contributed fundamentally to the breadth, depth, and pace of advances in diagnosing and treating disease and injury. But this progress has, in many instances, outstripped the health care system's capacity to know the circumstances under which a particular intervention is best applied. Without better information about the effectiveness of different treatment options, the resulting uncertainty can lead to the delivery of services that may be unnecessary, unproven, or even harmful. Other consequences of this gap between advancing treatment options and assessment capacity include a steady expansion in the national and personal costs of medical care, and a substantial growth in concern and distrust among physicians and patients alike. Accordingly, there is an acute need for better evidence to guide the decisions of patients and their caregivers on the approaches most appropriate to individual circumstances and preferences.

This need for a more systematic approach to evidence development and application, as well as the prospect of new ways of meeting the need, provided the back-drop for the IOM's 37th annual meeting, held in October 2007. The meeting drew heavily on discussions of the IOM's Roundtable on Evidence-Based Medicine. Through the Roundtable, the IOM has characterized evidence-based medicine to mean that *to the greatest extent possible, the decisions that shape the health and health care of Americans—by patients, providers, payers, and policy makers alike—will be grounded on a reliable evidence base, will account appropriately for individual variation in patient needs, and will support the generation of new insights on clinical effectiveness.* Evidence is generally considered to be information from clinical experience that has met some established test of validity, and the appropriate standard is determined according to the requirements of the intervention and clinical circumstance.

Evidence-Based Medicine and the Changing Nature of Health Care: Meeting Summary (2008) captures discussions at the 2007 IOM annual meeting on a range of issues—highlighting both challenges and opportunities to developing the health care system centered on the generation and application of evidence as a natural outcome of the care process. Discussion focused on four themes: the forces driving the need for better medical evidence; the challenges with which patients and providers must contend; the need to transform the speed and reliability of new medical evidence; and the legislative and policy changes that would enable an evidence-based health care system.

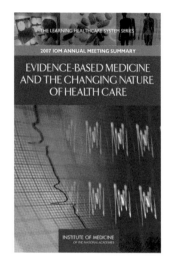

The report details a number of issues driving the need for a more central focus on evidence in health care. One underlying motif, for example, is the increasing complexity of health care. New pharmaceuticals, medical devices, technologies, and predictive data offer much promise for improving health care, but they also introduce a measure of uncertainty that requires changes on the parts of both caregivers and their patients.

Another frequent observation is that the current health care system is not designed to deliver value—a situation that leads to excessive medical spending, often on interventions of no clinical benefit. Unjustified discrepancies in care patterns also occur frequently. The intensity of health care services delivered for similar conditions varies significantly across geographic regions, particularly in areas that require discretionary decision making. However, the higher spending regions often do not deliver better quality care, and hence offer substantial opportunity for reduced spending without sacrificing health outcomes. Opportunities exist to eliminate wasteful spending with no reduction in health care, as well as to improve the overall health outcomes, but agreement is needed both on what constitutes best care and on what constitutes value in health care.

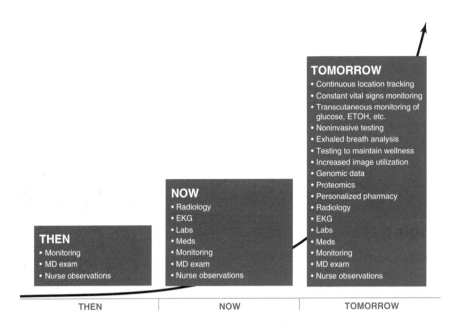

Data advances in medicine.

SOURCE: Evidence-Based Medicine and the Changing Nature of Health Care: Meeting Summary, p. 116.

These challenges illustrate the pressing need for more and better evidence development. Practice-based research approaches will help determine the effectiveness of new medical interventions and ways in which health care is delivered. Information technology offers additional promise to bring research closer to practice. Electronic medical records and clinical data registries, for example, offer tremendous potential both to generate new evidence and to augment randomized clinical trials. Capitalizing on such rewards will require addressing privacy and proprietary issues that now limit data access and sharing.

With the increasing complexity of care, and the need and demand for more patient involvement, the traditional "physician-as-sole-authority" model will need to adapt to support patients as integral partners in medical decisions.

Shifting to a culture of evidence-driven health care—what some observers call a "culture that learns"—will require health care providers and patients to support systems and procedures that foster the generation and application of evidence. Achieving such changes will mean developing new models of patient–provider partnerships. With the increasing complexity of care, and the need and demand for more patient involvement, the traditional "physician-as-sole-authority" model will need to adapt to support patients as integral partners in medical decisions.

As a foundation for these necessary changes, leadership promoting a focus on evidence in health care will need to stem from every quarter, with the public and private sectors working together, and with policy makers, providers, patients, insurers, and other stakeholders actively engaged in the steps toward change.

Gauging the nation's health

In order to understand how to improve the collective health of everyone in the United States, it is important first to understand the most significant factors that contribute to health and the effects of health care. At the request of the nonprofit group State of the USA, an IOM study committee has provided detailed guidance for producing just such a yardstick.

Clearly, no single measure can possibly capture the health of the nation. Thus, *State of the USA Health Indicators: Letter Report* (2008) lists 20 factors key to determining overall health and well-being. The indicators—each backed by a substantial body of high-quality data—fall into three general categories: health outcomes, health-related behaviors, and health systems performance. Health outcomes cover factors such as life expectancy at birth, infant mortality, injury-related mortality, and the prevalence of chronic diseases and psychological distress. Behavioral factors include both healthful activities, such as engaging regularly in at least moderate physical exercise, and harmful behaviors, such as smoking, drinking to excess, or being obese. Factors related to the performance of health systems include per-capita spending on care, pervasiveness of insurance coverage among populations, and rates of childhood immunization and adult preventative services, among others.

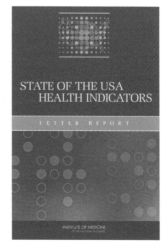

State of the USA is incorporating detailed information about these various measures into a new interactive website that anyone can use to

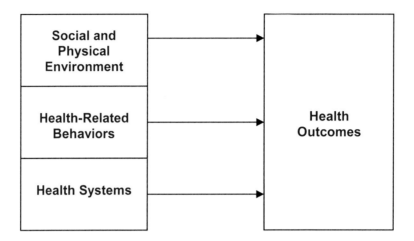

Framework for health and health care indicator development.

SOURCE: State of the USA Health Indicators: Letter Report, p. 5.

learn about critical health issues. They also will be able to track the nation's progress—or the progress of a particular geographic region—in improving the health of its population (or subpopulations) and gauge changes in the effectiveness of public health and care systems. Until now, only experts with the technological capability to search arcane data had the capacity for this kind of examination. As the nation moves increasingly toward "patient-centered medicine," in which patients play an active role in their treatment regimens, it will be important to develop effective ways to boost public knowledge about health issues. Certainly, technology is changing the game, allowing individuals to gather information directly and to use this information toward improving health—not only their own, but also the health of their community and of their country.

Meeting the Unique Health Needs of Women and Children

Women's health needs differ from those of men. Likewise, children are not simply miniature adults. A woman's body differs critically from a man's in both structure and function, and a child's body doesn't fully mimic an adult's. Each group's brain functions differently and responds in different ways to even the same stimuli. Each group often processes medications differently. And, of course, men, women, and children interact with the larger world and are affected by events in different ways.

Women and children have been labeled by some observers as the "unequal majority" in health and health care. Historically, the bulk of health studies have used adult men, with researchers and physicians left to infer how the studies apply to women and children. The conditions and needs of women and children, in large measure, have too frequently been set aside.

The Institute of Medicine (IOM) is working to ensure the health of the nation's women and children by focusing on their respective circumstances, including subject areas drawn from biological, environmental, social, clinical, and legal realms, among others. Studies consider a range of diverse issues that directly affect the health of individuals and their families or affect social programs that, in turn, contribute to the well-being of large groups of people.

Improving women's health during pregnancy

One question the IOM recently revisited is how much weight a pregnant woman should gain to protect both her health and the health of the developing fetus. Two decades ago, the IOM recommended guidelines, since widely adopted, for weight gain during pregnancy. But more research has been conducted on this subject, and over the past 20 years, there have been

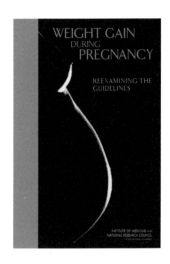

dramatic changes nationally in the diversity and health status of women having babies. Notably, women now tend to be older when they become pregnant, and they tend to be heavier, often entering pregnancy overweight or obese. Such changes may carry added health risks.

The IOM, with support from a number of government agencies and private organizations, has reviewed this changed landscape. The resulting report, *Weight Gain During Pregnancy: Reexamining the Guidelines* (2009), offers a set of recommendations—and some specific tools—that, if fully implemented, represent an important change in the care provided to women of child-bearing age. The new guidelines consider not only the welfare of the infant, as the original guidelines did, but also the health of the mother.

Among its core findings, the report says that women should have a normal body mass index (a measure of body fat based on weight and

New Recommendations for Total and Rate of Weight Gain During Pregnancy, by Prepregnancy Body Mass Index (BMI)

Prepregnancy BMI	Total Weight Gain		Rates of Weight Gain* 2nd and 3rd Trimester	
	Range in kg	Range in lbs	Mean (range) in kg/week	Mean (range) in lbs/week
Underweight (< 18.5 kg/m²)	12.5–18	28–40	0.51 (0.44–0.58)	1 (1–1.3)
Normal-weight (18.5–24.9 kg/m²)	11.5–16	25–35	0.42 (0.35–0.50)	1 (0.8–1)
Overweight (25.0–29.9 kg/m²)	7–11.5	15–25	0.28 (0.23–0.33)	0.6 (0.5–0.7)
Obese (≥ 30.0 kg/m²)	5–9	11–20	0.22 (0.17–0.27)	0.5 (0.4–0.6)

*Calculations assume a 0.5–2 kg (1.1– 4.4 lbs) weight gain in the first trimester.

SOURCE: Weight Gain During Pregnancy: Reexamining the Guidelines, p. 254.

height) when they become pregnant, and that they should gain weight during their pregnancy within a fairly narrow range, based on their age, race or ethnicity, and various other factors that may affect pregnancy outcomes. Meeting these guidelines will require women and their care providers to work together, starting before conception, with counseling efforts, often including planning for preconception weight loss.

Notably, women now tend to be older when they become pregnant, and they tend to be heavier, often entering pregnancy overweight or obese. Such changes may carry added health risks.

The report calls on federal agencies, private voluntary organizations, and medical and public health organizations to adopt the new guidelines and publicize them to their members and to women of childbearing age.

Reviewing federal family planning programs

Family planning is known to help women—as well as men—maintain their reproductive health, and it also enables women to avoid unintended pregnancies and plan for pregnancies. Collectively, such benefits contribute to the well-being of individuals, families, and broader society. Even so, many low-income individuals find it difficult to pay for these services, highlighting the critical role played by the Title X Family Planning Program, the nation's only federal program, created in 1970, exclusively devoted to providing family planning services.

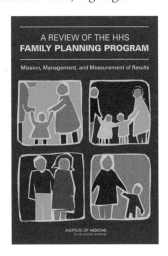

At the request of the Office of Family Planning, the agency within the U.S. Department of Health and Human Services (HHS) that administers the Title X Family Planning Program, the IOM conducted a comprehensive review of the program. The resulting report, *A Review of the HHS Family Planning Program: Mission, Management, and Measurement of Results* (2009), finds that the Title X program, in large measure, has successfully delivered critical services to those who have the most difficulty obtaining them. However, if the program is going to truly meet the needs of its targeted groups—low-income individuals and adolescents—several structural components need to be improved.

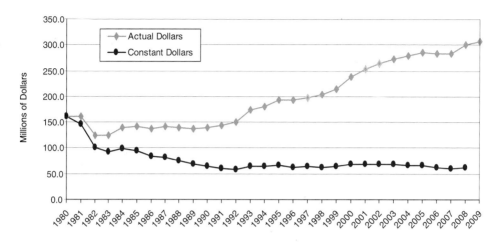

Estimated funding for Title X when adjusted for inflation, FY 1980–2009.

SOURCE: A Review of the HHS Family Planning Program: Mission, Management, and Measurement of Results, p. 111.

In particular, the Office of Family Planning lacks a clear process for establishing or revising program priorities and guidelines, and developing such a process is an important priority. The strategic plan must reflect the original mission of the Title X program and an understanding of its target population; incorporate lessons gained from the field of family planning and reproductive health; provide a vision for coordination, leadership, and evaluation; address the family planning needs of individuals over the full reproductive lifespan; and be firmly grounded in high-quality evidence.

Reducing depression's grip on parents and children

Depression affects millions of U.S. adults over their lifetime, many of whom are parents with children. The burden of depression and the barriers to quality of care for depressed adults are increasingly well understood, but the ways in which depression affects parenting—and, in turn, children's health and psychological functioning—are often ignored.

To illuminate this problem and identify solutions, the IOM and National Research Council convened a committee to consider the identification, prevention, and treatment of parental depression, along with its interaction with parenting practices, and its effects on children and families. The resulting report, *Depression in Parents, Parenting, and Children: Opportunities to Improve Identification, Treatment, and Prevention* (2009), finds that parental depression is prevalent, but a comprehensive strategy to treat the depressed adults and to prevent problems in their children is absent.

The report concludes that national leadership, interagency collaboration, federal–state cooperation, and government collaboration with the private sector are needed to support the development and evaluation of a framework that integrates health, mental health, public health, and parenting in a life-course framework, from pregnancy through adolescence. Federal and state governments also should provide additional support for public and professional education, training, infrastructure development, and implementation efforts to improve the quality of services for affected families and vulnerable children. Likewise, more funding is needed for research, data collection, and evaluation efforts that might lead to improved prevention and treatment services for this population.

Improving adolescent health services

Nearly 42 million adolescents aged 10 to 19 live in the United States, and most of them are healthy. But all too frequently, young people engage in risky behavior, develop unhealthful habits, or have chronic conditions that can jeopardize both their immediate and long-term health and safety. The three leading causes of death in adolescents—motor vehicle crashes, homicide, and suicide—all are tied to risky and unhealthful behaviors. As well, adolescence is a critical period for developing positive habits and skills that create a strong foundation for healthful lifestyles and behavior over the full lifespan. Growing up without having developed these habits can be detrimental to an adult's health and well-being.

The system should foster coordination between primary and specialty care, and it should enable primary care providers to more easily reach and follow adolescents through "safety net" settings such as hospitals and community health centers.

The U.S. health care system has a potentially key role in promoting adolescent health. But an IOM study, conducted with the National Research Council and funded by The Atlantic Philanthropies, finds that the system is failing in that role. The study report, *Adolescent Health Services: Missing Opportunities* (2009), says that services often are fragmented and poorly coordinated across various settings, resulting in gaps in care in reaching all of the nation's adolescents during this criti-

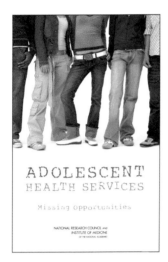

ADOLESCENT
HEALTH SERVICES

Missing Opportunities

NATIONAL RESEARCH COUNCIL and
INSTITUTE OF MEDICINE
OF THE NATIONAL ACADEMIES

cal period. Many health services also are poorly equipped to meet the disease prevention, health promotion, and behavioral needs of adolescents, and many care providers lack the necessary skills to interact appropriately and effectively with this age group. Moreover, large numbers of adolescents are uninsured or have inadequate health insurance, and so are unable to access care, even where available.

As a blueprint for action, the report highlights critical health needs of adolescents, details promising models of health services, and identifies components of care that could strengthen and improve health services for adolescents and contribute to healthy adolescent development. Among specific steps, federal and state agencies, private foundations, and insurers should work together to develop a care system that improves services for all ado-

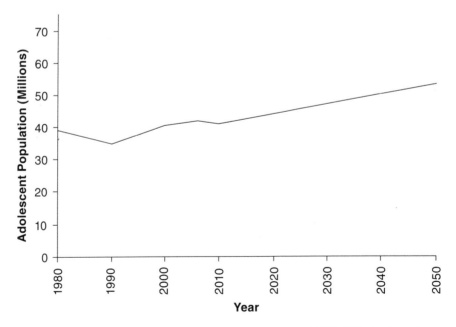

Growth in the adolescent population, aged 10 to 19, 1980–2006 and 2006–2050 (projected).

SOURCE: Adolescent Health Services: Missing Opportunities, p. 32.

lescents. The system should foster coordination between primary and specialty care, and it should enable primary care providers to more easily reach and follow adolescents through "safety net" settings such as hospitals and community health centers.

Training health professionals will be critical as well. At all levels of professional education, providers should receive comprehensive education about adolescents' health problems and effective ways to treat their diseases and promote healthful behaviors. Furthermore, confidentiality should be protected for adolescents receiving care. They should give their own consent before receiving care and before their health information is shared with others, even their parents. Finally, the more than 5 million medically uninsured adolescents indicate a clear need for federal and state policy makers to develop strategies to ensure that all adolescents have comprehensive, continuous health insurance coverage.

Improving mental, emotional, and behavioral health among young people

Among the most dangerous risks to the health and well-being of young people are depression, conduct disorder, substance abuse, and similar disorders. They are as commonplace today as are fractured limbs—not inevitable, but not at all unusual—and they often carry over into adulthood. Almost one in five young people has such a disorder, or even multiple disorders, at any given time. Among adults, half of all mental, emotional, and behavioral disorders were first diagnosed by age 14 and three-fourths by age 24. In addition to their health toll, the disorders exact high economic and psychosocial costs, not only for the young people, but also for their families, schools, and communities. The price tag for treatment services and lost productivity runs an estimated $247 billion annually.

Among adults, half of all mental, emotional, and behavioral disorders were first diagnosed by age 14 and three-fourths by age 24.

The good news is that much is known about how to prevent these disorders before they occur. Risk factors are well established, preventive interventions are available, and the first symptoms typically precede a disorder by 2 to 4 years. Yet the nation's health system approach largely has been to wait to act until a disorder is well established and has already done considerable harm. All too often, opportunities are missed to use evidence-based approaches to prevent the occurrence of mental, emotional, or behavioral disorders; establish building blocks for healthy development in all young people; and limit the environmental exposures that increase risk—approaches likely to be far more cost effective in addressing such disorders in the long run.

Preventing Mental, Emotional, and Behavioral Disorders Among Young People

Progress and Possibilities

NATIONAL RESEARCH COUNCIL and INSTITUTE OF MEDICINE OF THE NATIONAL ACADEMIES

To help in building a better health system, the National Research Council and the IOM recently reviewed the research on the prevention of mental disorders and substance abuse among young people. *Preventing Mental, Emotional, and Behavioral Disorders Among Young People: Progress and Possibilities* (2009) recommends a variety of strategies to improve the psychological and emotional well-being of this target population. The report updates a key 1994 IOM report, *Reducing Risks for Mental Disorders*, focusing special attention on the research and program experiences that have emerged since that time.

The report describes the value of a number of prevention strategies, including:

- *Strengthening families* by targeting problems such as substance use or aggressive behavior; teaching effective parenting skills; improving communication; and helping families deal with disruptions (such as divorce) or adversities (such as parental mental illness or poverty).

- *Strengthening individuals* by building resilience and skills and improving cognitive processes and behaviors.

- *Preventing specific disorders*, such as anxiety or depression, by screening individuals at risk and offering cognitive training or other preventive interventions.

- *Promoting mental health in schools* by offering support to children encountering serious stresses; modifying the school environment to promote healthful social behavior; developing students' skills at decision making, self-awareness, and conducting relationships; and targeting violence, aggressive behavior, and substance use.

- *Promoting mental health in communities* by supporting programs designed to foster healthful social behavior; teach coping skills; and target modifiable lifestyle factors, such as sleep, diet, activity and

physical fitness, exposure to sunshine and light, and television view-
ing, that can affect behavior and emotional health.

How best to capitalize on such strategies? Many providers and agencies are responsible for the care, protection, or support of young people:
the child welfare, education, and juvenile justice systems, as well as medical and mental health care providers and community organizations. Yet
resources within these agencies are scattered, not coordinated, and often
do not effectively support prevention programs or policies. To stitch
together such patchwork national leadership is necessary to make systematic prevention efforts a high priority in the health care system as well as an
integral component of local, state, and federal programs that serve young
people and families.

Prevalence Estimates of Mental, Emotional, and Behavioral Disorders in Young People

Diagnosis or Diagnostic Group (N of studies contributing to estimate)	Preva-lence (%)	Standard Error (%)	Lower 95%	Upper 95%
One or more disorders (44)	17.0	1.3	14.4	19.6
Unipolar depression (31)	5.2	0.7	4.0	7.0
Any anxiety disorder (29)	8.0	1.0	6.2	10.3
Generalized anxiety disorder (17)	1.3	0.3	0.9	2.0
Separation anxiety disorder (17)	4.1	0.9	2.6	9.4
Social phobia (15)	4.2	1.1	2.4	7.3
Specific phobia (13)	3.7	1.3	1.7	7.7
Panic (12)	0.7	0.2	0.3	1.5
Posttraumatic stress disorder (7)	0.6	0.2	0.3	1.1
Attention deficit hyperactivity disorder (34)	4.5	0.7	3.3	6.2
Any disruptive behavior disorder (23)	6.1	0.5	5.4	7.3
Conduct disorder (28)	3.5	0.5	2.7	4.7
Oppositional defiant disorder (21)	2.8	0.4	2.1	3.7
Substance use disorder (12)	10.3	2.2	6.3	16.2
Alcohol use disorder (9)	4.3	1.4	2.1	8.9

NOTE: The prevalence estimates from each study were transformed to logit scale and their
standard errors computed using the available information about the sample size and prevalences.
Using weights inversely proportional to estimated variances, weighted linear regression models
were fit in SAS, using PROC GENMOD with study as a fixed effect (class variable). The overall
estimate (on the logit scale) and its standard error were then used to recompute the overall prevalence and its standard error using the delta method.

SOURCE: Preventing Mental, Emotional, and Behavioral Disorders Among Young People: Progress
and Possibilities, p. 43.

Among specific steps, the committee recommends that the White House develop an interdepartmental strategy that identifies specific prevention goals, directs multiple federal agency resources toward these goals, and provides guidance to state and local partners. In turn, governments at all levels should increase their investments in prevention and promotion, including setting aside resources for evidence-based prevention in mental health service programs and funding proven prevention approaches by school systems. Adequately funded state and local systems should craft partnerships among families, schools, courts, health care providers, and local programs to create coordinated approaches that support healthy development.

Public and private organizations also should increase efforts to beef up the professional workforce by fostering development of training programs and prevention standards across disciplines, including health, education, and social work. On a broader stage, a range of public and private organizations should join in promoting public education, making use of mass media and the Internet to share information about risk factors and available interventions, as well as to reduce the stigma often associated with mental, emotional, and behavioral disorders.

Assessing early childhood enrichment programs

In the nation's increasing drive to improve young children's education and development, a host of public and private organizations have developed programs to enhance the school readiness of all children, especially those from economically disadvantaged homes and communities, those with special needs, and those who learn English as a second language. These early childhood education and child care programs, such as Head Start, run by the HHS, are designed to enhance social, language, and academic skills, as well as to identify children with developmental problems so they can be given appropriate interventions.

At the same time, early childhood education and intervention programs are increasingly being asked to prove their worth. At the request of Congress, the National Research Council, with the assistance of the IOM and funding from HHS, considered how to identify important developmental outcomes of preschool children—from birth to age 5—and how best to assess them in preschools, child care settings, and other early childhood programs. The resulting report, *Early Childhood Assessment: Why, What, and How* (2008), concludes that well-planned assessments can inform teaching and efforts to improve programs and can contribute to better outcomes for children. Poor assessments or misuse of the results, however, can harm both children and programs.

The report emphasizes the need to view assessment as part of a broader system of early childhood interventions. It offers a set of principles to guide the design, implementation, and use of assessments in early childhood settings. As an overarching rule, good assessments must be designed for specific purposes, and their aims should not be mixed. For example, the assessment of a program's performance should not be used to judge the performance of an individual child. The purpose of any assessment should be made explicit and public in advance, and it should be conducted within a coherent system of health, educational, and family support services that promote optimal development for all children. System officials should provide clearly articulated standards for what children should learn and what constitutes a quality program.

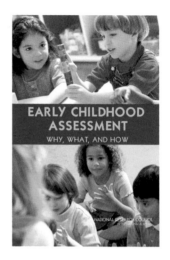

The report also pays attention to the limits of assessments and their possible adverse effects. On the practical side, some types of assessments may make children feel anxious, incompetent, or bored, while other types may constitute a burden on adults. Assessments also cost money, and they may deflect time and resources from instruction. Therefore it is important to ensure that the value of the information gathered through assessments outweighs any negative effects on adults or children and that it merits the investment of resources. Assessments done improperly also can lead to bad high-stakes decisions, all of which should be considered seriously.

The report calls for future research to improve the quality and suitability of developmental assessment across a wide array of purposes. For example, some assessment measures have been tested only with populations that do not represent the diversity of children enrolled in today's early childhood programs. Thus, care should be used in assessing the status or progress of young children with special needs and those for whom English is a second language, as many existing assessment tools have not demonstrated their validity for these groups.

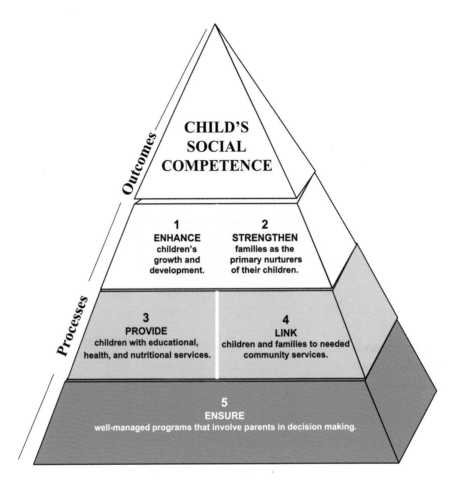

Head Start Program performance measures conceptual framework.

SOURCE: Early Childhood Assessment: Why, What, and How, p. 51.

Critiquing a national child health study research plan

As important as it is to evaluate children's developmental programs, it is similarly important to monitor the impact of a child's environment on his or her health. A variety of environmental influences are said to threaten children's health. Some are well known and widely studied. For example, a child who was exposed as a fetus to certain compounds, including lead and alcohol, often experiences a range of serious health problems. But there is considerable uncertainty about the relationship of other environmental factors to what often appear to be growing health problems among children, including asthma, autism, developmental disorders, obesity, and childhood cancers.

In response to both congressional and presidential initiatives, the Eunice Kennedy Shriver National Institute of Child Health and Human Development (NICHD), in cooperation with several other federal agencies, is undertaking the National Children's Study (NCS). The NCS will be the largest long-term study of environmental effects on children's health ever conducted in the United States. It proposes to examine the effects of environmental influences on the health and development of approximately 100,000 children nationwide, following them from before birth until age 21. Data will be gathered on an array of measures of biological, chemical, physical, genetic, social, cultural, geographical, and other factors in a child's environment that can affect health and development. The NCS proposes to examine many different exposures and establish—or rule out—relationships between them with many different outcomes. In archiving the data, the NCS is intended to provide a valuable resource for analyses conducted many years into the future.

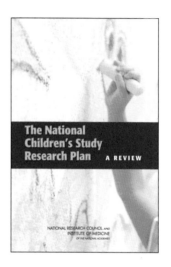

But how should the study be done? At the request of NICHD, the National Research Council and the IOM studied the proposed research plan to assess its scientific rigor and the extent to which the NCS is being carried out with methods, measures, and collection of data and specimens to maximize scientific yields. *The National Children's Study Research Plan: A Review* (2008) finds that overall, the NCS looks promising. As proposed, the resulting database should be valuable for investigating the various hypotheses about exposures and health effects described in the plan, as well as additional hypotheses that are likely to evolve as the study proceeds.

Among the plan's strengths, it would provide enough statistical power to examine many hypothesized relations that cannot be investigated with smaller samples. The data, gathered prospectively over the entire course of pregnancy, childhood, adolescence, and early adulthood, will enable exploration of many new relations between exposures and outcomes. For example, data will be collected in women from before they conceive and during the early stages of gestation, a period when certain environmental

A New Definition of Children's Health

The report of the Committee on Evaluation of Children's Health, *Children's Health, The Nation's Wealth* (National Research Council and Institute of Medicine, 2004), defines children's health as follows:

> Children's health is the extent to which individual children or groups of children are able or enabled to (a) develop and realize their potential, (b) satisfy their needs, and (c) develop the capacities that allow them to interact successfully with their biological, physical, and social environments.

This definition draws upon an explanation from the World Health Organization that health is a state of complete physical, mental, and social well-being, not merely the absence of disease or infirmity; a collaborative effort of the European Union Health Monitoring Programme to develop the Child Health Indicators of Life and Development model; the positive health principles embraced by the Ottawa Charter for Health Promotion (1986); and the research literature cited in the report.

Key features of the new definition of children's health include three distinct but related domains:

- health conditions, "a domain that deals with disorders or illnesses";

- functioning, "which focuses on the manifestations of individual health in daily life"; and

exposures may prove to be critically important. Additionally, the array of measures to be documented will permit investigation of relationships that have not previously been studied.

But the NCS also has some important weaknesses and shortcomings that may diminish the study's value. First, the study is being implemented without sufficient pilot testing. The study design is extremely complex in

- health potential, "which captures the development of health assets that indicate positive aspects—competence, capacity, and developmental potential."

The report describes these domains in detail and also describes ways to measure not only aspects of each domain, but also the influences on children's health, which are defined to include:

- Children's biology

- Children's behavior

- Physical environment
  - o   Prenatal exposures
  - o   Childhood exposures
  - o   Home, school, and work settings
  - o   Child injury and the provision of safe environments
  - o   The built environment

- Social environment
  - o   Family
  - o   Community
  - o   Culture
  - o   Discrimination

- Services

- Policy

SOURCE: The National Children's Study Research Plan: A Review, p. 45.

terms of identifying subjects, enlisting their enrollment and continued participation, administering the large number of survey and clinical instruments, and managing huge databases generated by disparate organizations. In addition, there are various technical questions concerning the kinds of measurement instruments to be used and the timing of their application. Such concerns could be addressed during an expanded pilot phase to great benefit.

Another potential trouble spot is the plan's failure to prepare adequately for disclosure of risk to participants. As soon as data collection begins, the NCS will face questions about the circumstances under which information about a child's health and development, as well as his or her exposure to toxic agents, should be conveyed to participants and their parents. The study calls for providing information on conditions that are "clinically relevant and actionable," but this category needs to be better defined and made operational. Similarly, there is insufficient detail in the plan about how decisions will be made about what to disclose. Some of the decisions—for example, regarding transmitting information about fetal defects encountered through ultrasounds—urgently need to be made.

Improving the Nation's Health Care System

The United States currently spends more than $2.2 trillion annually on health care expenses, including costs borne by the government, the private sector, and individuals. In 2007, the latest year for which data are available, the nation spent on health care 16 percent of its gross domestic product, the broadest measure of economic output—a level higher than any other developed nation. Many observers argue that with this level of investment, the nation should be able to provide all of its residents with quality health care. Yet the health care system falls well short of that goal. Nearly every component of the system costs too much to operate, and the various components too often fail to work together, with the whole system becoming less than the sum of its parts. But perhaps the system's overarching flaw is that it provides many patients with less-than-optimal care or, in some cases, no care at all. Such concerns are driving interest in health care reform from both sides of the political aisle.

The Institute of Medicine (IOM) seeks ways to help reinvigorate the health care system every year. Studies range from crafting blueprints for major system overhauls to offering guidance for how health care professionals should provide care to patients, to studies on development of policies and technologies that reduce the effects of disabilities.

Creating a health care system that works well

The nation's health care system is complex almost beyond description, with payers, providers, regulators, and patients interacting in myriad ways.

Across every sector of the system, opportunities exist to streamline operations and improve patient care.

Coping with an aging population

The nation is rapidly growing older. By 2030, the number of adults aged 65 and older will almost double, placing accelerating demands on the nation's health care system. Older adults rely on health care services far more than other segments of the population. Additionally, this cohort of elderly people will be the most diverse the nation has ever seen, with greater education,

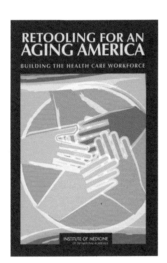

increased longevity, widely dispersed families, and more racial and ethnic diversity, making their needs much different than previous generations.

With support from a number of private organizations, the IOM examined what this explosion of older people will mean for the nation and how it can prepare to meet the challenges certain to arise. *Retooling for an Aging America: Building the Health Care Workforce* (2008) finds that the current workforce is too small and woefully unprepared to provide an adequate level of high-quality care to this growing population group, and it calls for a series of bold initiatives—starting immediately.

Among the initiatives, a national effort is needed to train all health care providers in the basics of geriatric care. Such training may be undertaken in health professional schools and health care training programs or through other means. A national push also is needed to better prepare family members and other informal caregivers to tend to older people, as well as to prepare these individuals to take more active roles in their own care. To foster such efforts, Medicare, Medicaid, and other health plans should pay more for the services of geriatric specialists and direct-care workers to attract more health professionals and to staunch turnover among care aides, many of whom earn wages below the poverty level.

Governments at all levels, along with a spectrum of health care organizations, need to do more to disseminate innovative models of care delivery that have proved efficient and cost effective for older adults. Diffusion of such models has been minimal, often because current financing systems do not provide payment for features such as patient education, care

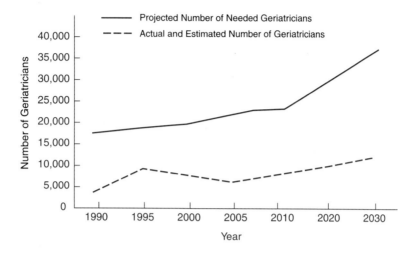

Projected number of needed geriatricians.

SOURCE: Retooling for an Aging America: Building the Health Care Workforce, p. 20.

coordination, and interdisciplinary care. Because no single model of care will be sufficient to meet the needs of all older adults, Congress and public and private foundations should significantly increase support for research and programs that promote the development of additional innovative care models, especially in areas where effective delivery models are lacking, such as in preventive and palliative care.

The IOM accompanied the report's release with an intensive communication outreach effort, which included, among other activities, three symposia held across the country to discuss various aspects of the report and extensive briefings of congressional leaders.

As a direct result, in December 2008, Senator Herb Kohl (D-WI) and Representative Jan Schakowsky (D-IL) jointly introduced the Retooling the Health Care Workforce for an Aging America Act, which

> **By 2030, the number of adults aged 65 and older will almost double, placing accelerating demands on the nation's health care system.**

incorporates the report's recommendations. According to its sponsors, the bill "aims to expand education and training opportunities in geriatrics and long-term care for licensed health professionals, direct-care workers, and family caregivers." Both the Senate and House bills were referred to Committee in early 2009.

In another of the report's ripple effects, a group of national organizations representing older adults, health care professionals, direct-care workers, and family caregivers joined together to form the Eldercare Workforce Alliance. Now with 29 members, the alliance is working to implement many of the IOM's recommendations.

Restructuring medical resident training

Among the many recommendations aimed at preparing the nation for an aging baby boomer population is a clear need to address the training of future doctors. In addition to the great need to train geriatric specialists, however, the nation also must address how to better train all medical residents. As an important part of their training, recent medical school graduates must serve a residency to prepare them to practice medicine independently. During the 3 to 7 years of this training, residents often work long hours with limited time off to prevent acute and chronic sleep deprivation. Some observers argue that such duty hours may unduly fatigue residents and lead to increased risk of medical errors and accidents. Many medical educators, on the other hand, maintain that extensive duty hours are essential to provide

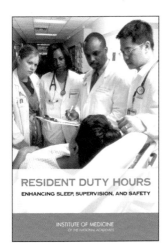

RESIDENT DUTY HOURS
ENHANCING SLEEP, SUPERVISION, AND SAFETY

INSTITUTE OF MEDICINE
OF THE NATIONAL ACADEMIES

residents with the educational experiences necessary to become competent in the complexities of diagnosing and treating patients.

At the request of Congress and with support from the U.S. Agency for Healthcare Research and Quality, the IOM evaluated current evidence on this thorny issue. *Resident Duty Hours: Enhancing Sleep, Supervision, and Safety* (2009) finds considerable scientific evidence that the amount of duty hours permitted in current resident work schedules can result in fatigue and the chance of fatigue-related medical errors, and that adjustments to the duty hour limits are needed. The report does not recommend reducing the total residents' work hours from the maximum average of 80 per week now allowed. Rather, the report recommends that the Accreditation Council for Graduate Medical Education, which sets the standard, reduce the maximum number of hours that residents can work without time for sleep to 16, down from 30 hours; increase the number of days residents must have off; and restrict moonlighting during residents' off-hours, among other changes. The report also

Comparison of IOM Committee Adjustments to the Accreditation Council for Graduate Medical Education's (ACGME's) Current Duty Hour Limits

	2003 ACGME Duty Hour Limits	IOM Recommendation
Maximum hours of work per week	80 hours, averaged over 4 weeks	No change
Maximum shift length	30 hours (admitting patients up to 24 hours then 6 additional hours for transitional and educational activities)	• 30 hours (admitting patients for up to 16 hours, plus 5-hour protected sleep period between 10 p.m. and 8 a.m. with the remaining hours for transition and educational activities) • 16 hours with no protected sleep period
Maximum in-hospital on-call frequency	Every third night, on average	Every third night, no averaging
Minimum time off between scheduled shifts	10 hours after shift length	• 10 hours after day shift • 12 hours after night shift • 14 hours after any extended duty period of 30 hours and not return until 6 a.m. of next day
Maximum frequency of in-hospital night shifts	Not addressed	4 night maximum; 48 hours off after 3 or 4 nights of consecutive duty
Mandatory time off duty	• 4 days off per month • 1 day (24 hours) off per week, averaged over 4 weeks	• 5 days off per month • 1 day (24 hours) off per week, no averaging • One 48-hour period off per month
Moonlighting	Internal moonlighting is counted against 80-hour weekly limit	• Internal and external moonlighting is counted against 80-hour weekly limit • All other duty hour limits apply to moonlighting in combination with scheduled work
Limit on hours for exceptions	88 hours for select programs with a sound educational rationale	No change
Emergency room limits	12-hour shift limit, at least an equivalent period of time off between shifts; 60-hour workweek with additional 12 hours for education	No change

SOURCE: Resident Duty Hours: Enhancing Sleep, Supervision, and Safety, p. 13.

calls for greater supervision of residents by experienced physicians, limits on patient caseloads based on residents' levels of experience and specialties, and better patient handover procedures, as well as an overlap in schedules during shift changes to reduce the chances for error during the handover of patients from one doctor to another.

During the 3 to 7 years of this training, residents often work long hours with limited time off to prevent acute and chronic sleep deprivation.

Financial costs and an insufficient health care workforce are the biggest barriers to revising resident hours. Accordingly, all financial stakeholders in graduate medical education should provide additional funding for teaching hospitals to cover the additional costs—an estimated $1.7 billion annually—associated with shifting some work from current residents to other health care personnel or additional residents. At the same time, productivity and quality gains among residents may help offset these costs. For example, a previous IOM report, *Preventing Medical Errors* (2006), found that the extra medical costs of treating drug-related injuries occurring in hospitals nationwide conservatively amount to $3.5 billion a year.

Improving cancer care

With nearly 1.5 million new cases of cancer expected to be diagnosed in America in 2009, the effect of the disease on the nation can hardly be

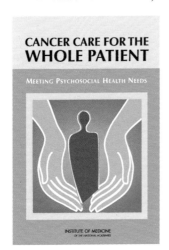

overstated. Cancer impacts not only patients and their families, but also the health care workforce, and it is connected to many other challenges, from research strategies to end-of-life care, that confront society. Patients are living longer thanks to cancer care today that provides state-of-the-science biomedical treatment. But the treatments often fail to address the psychological and social problems associated with the illness—or with the treatments themselves—and patients and their families suffer in various ways.

At the request of the National Institutes of Health (NIH), the IOM took an in-depth look at how cancer patients might be better served. *Cancer Care for the Whole Patient: Meeting Psychosocial Health Needs* (2007) concludes that care that focuses solely on eradicating tumors without taking account of the patient's general well-being falls short of quality care. Such incomplete care may increase a patient's suffering and compromise his or her ability to follow through on treatment. As a remedy, the nation should adopt a new standard of care under which all oncology care providers would systematically screen patients for distress and other problems; connect patients with health care or service providers who have resources to meet these needs and coordinate care with these professionals; and periodically reevaluate patients to determine if any changes in care are indicated.

As a guide to achieving this standard, the report recommends a set of 10 actions that should be taken by oncology providers, health policy makers, educators, health insurers, health plans, quality oversight organizations, researchers and research sponsors, and consumer advocates. As one step,

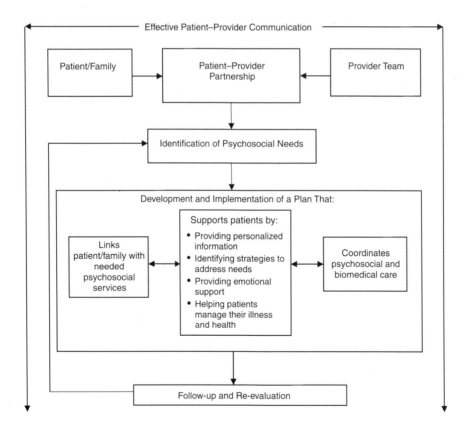

Model for the delivery of psychosocial health services.

SOURCE: Cancer Care for the Whole Patient: Meeting Psychosocial Health Needs, p. 8.

group purchasers of health care—Medicare, Medicaid, and employers—and health insurance plans should assess how psychosocial care is addressed in their agreements with each other and with health care providers, and then determine the adequacy of payment rates, adjusting them as necessary. In addition, a number of government and private organizations can encourage cancer care providers to adhere to the new standard. For example, the National Cancer Institute (NCI), as the nation's leader in developing better approaches to cancer care, could include requirements for meeting psychosocial health needs in its protocols and programs. Standard-setting organizations, such as the National Comprehensive Cancer Network and the American College of Surgeons' Commission on Cancer, also could incorporate the new standard and its components into their own standards.

Leaders in the field were listening. At a congressional briefing in March 2008, a high-ranking official at the NCI reported that his agency has taken numerous steps to implement some of the report's recommendations. For example, the Institute is continuing to fund "centers of excellence" in patient-centered communications; providing community cancer centers with support to conduct patient experience surveys; and pursuing a number of projects, often in collaboration with other agencies, to improve measurement of "whole patient" outcomes, with the end goal being development of a national monitoring and surveillance system.

Reducing conflicts of interest in medical research

In cancer as well as many other areas of medicine, collaborations of physicians and researchers with industry can provide valuable benefits to society, particularly in the translation of basic scientific discoveries to new therapies and products. But financial ties between medicine and industry may create conflicts of interest that put at risk the integrity of medical research, the objectivity of professional education, the quality of patient care, the soundness of clinical practice guidelines, and the public's trust in medicine.

... the report notes that if industry and the medical community fail to strengthen their conflict-of-interest policies, practices, and enforcement, more policy makers may turn to legislative solutions, as officials in some states already have.

With support from the NIH and several private foundations, the IOM took a comprehensive look at the risks of—and possible solutions to—such conflicts. *Conflict of Interest in Medical Research, Education, and Practice* (2009) offers principles to inform the design of policies to identify, limit, and manage conflicts of interest without damaging constructive collaboration with industry. It calls for both short-term actions and long-term commitments by institutions and individuals, including leaders of academic medical centers, professional societies, patient advocacy groups, government agencies, and companies that manufacture drugs and medical devices.

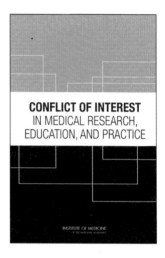

Among key steps, researchers, medical school faculty, and private-practice doctors should forgo gifts of any amount from medical companies and should decline to publish or present material ghostwritten or otherwise controlled by industry. Consulting arrangements should be limited to legitimate expert services spelled out in formal contracts and paid for at a fair market rate. Physicians should limit their interactions with company sales representatives and use free drug samples only for patients who cannot afford medications. At a broader level, all academic medical centers, journals, professional societies, and other entities engaged in health research, education, clinical care, and development of practice guidelines should establish or strengthen conflict-of-interest policies.

On the other side of the coin, Congress should require pharmaceutical, biotechnology, and device firms to report through a public website the payments they make to doctors, researchers, academic health centers, professional societies, patient advocacy groups, and others involved in medicine. Such a public record could serve as a deterrent to inappropriate relationships and undue industry influence, and would provide medical institutions with a way to verify the accuracy of information that physicians, researchers, and senior officials have disclosed to them.

Although the report calls for some new legislation and regulations, it emphasizes the role of voluntary efforts by the various stakeholders, stressing that voluntary action is more likely to reinforce professional values and foster policies that minimize unintended consequences and administrative burdens. But the report notes that if industry and the medical community fail to strengthen their conflict-of-interest policies, practices, and enforcement, more policy makers may turn to legislative solutions, as officials in some states already have.

Conflict of Interest Report Recommendations in Overview

Recommendation Number and Topic	Primary Actors
General policy	
3.1 Adopt and implement conflict of interest policies	Institutions that carry out medical research and education, clinical care, and clinical practice guideline development
3.2 Strengthen disclosure policies	Institutions that carry out medical research and education, clinical care, and clinical practice guideline development
3.3 Standardize disclosure content and formats	Institutions that carry out medical research and education, clinical care, and clinical practice guideline development and other interested organizations (e.g., accrediting bodies, health insurers, consumer groups, and government agencies)
3.4 Create a national program for the reporting of company payments	U.S. Congress; pharmaceutical, medical device, and biotechnology companies
Medical research	
4.1 Restrict participation of researchers with conflicts of interest in research with human participants	Academic medical centers and other research institutions; medical researchers
Medical education	
5.1 Reform relationships with industry in medical education	Academic medical centers and teaching hospitals; faculty, students, residents, and fellows
5.2 Provide education on conflict of interest	Academic medical centers and teaching hospitals; professional societies
5.3 Reform financing system for continuing medical education	Organizations that created the accrediting program for continuing medical education and other organizations interested in high-quality, objective education
Medical practice	
6.1 Reform financial relationships with industry for community physicians	Community physicians; professional societies; hospitals and other health care providers
6.2 Reform industry interactions with physicians	Pharmaceutical, medical device, and biotechnology companies

Continued

Recommendation Number and Topic	Primary Actors
Clinical practice guidelines	
7.1 Restrict industry funding and conflicts in clinical practice guideline development	Institutions that develop clinical practice guidelines
7.2 Create incentives for reducing conflicts in clinical practice guideline development	Accrediting and certification bodies, formulary committees, health insurers, public agencies, and other organizations with an interest in objective, evidence-based clinical practice guidelines
Institutional conflict of interest policies	
8.1 Create board-level responsibility for institutional conflicts of interest	Institutions that carry out medical research and education, clinical care, and clinical practice guideline development
8.2 Revise Public Health Service regulations to require policies on institutional conflicts of interest	National Institutes of Health
Supporting organizations	
9.1 Provide additional incentives for institutions to adopt and implement policies	Oversight bodies and other groups that have a strong interest in or reliance on medical research, education, clinical care, and practice guideline development
9.2 Develop research agenda on conflict of interest	NIH, Agency for Healthcare Research and Quality, and other agencies of the U.S. Department of Health and Human Services

SOURCE: Conflict of Interest in Medical Research, Education, and Practice, p. 16.

Advancing the national health agenda

As policy makers work to create a blueprint for health care in the years ahead, they must consider both establishing new policies and programs and reforming those that do not function well. A recent IOM report, *HHS in the 21st Century: Charting a New Course for a Healthier America* (2008), described earlier in this book, suggests ways in which the U.S. Department of Health and Human Services (HHS) can be improved. Subsequent work by the IOM discusses other strategies for improving the nation's care.

As part of a universal effort to bring down health care costs in the United States while improving the quality of the care provided, Congress requested in the American Recovery and Reinvestment Act that the IOM conduct a study to determine the appropriate national priorities for comparative effectiveness research.

The medical field depends on the trust placed by patients in their doctors and in their doctors' advice about treatment and care. Yet often, physicians and patients must make decisions in the absence of complete information because the evidence is lacking for the effectiveness of one approach compared to another. Comparative effectiveness research offers the opportunity to demonstrate the effectiveness of one strategy over another for a certain condition, enabling doctors and patients to make smarter health decisions founded in sound scientific evidence. One of the fundamental aims of comparative effectiveness research is to help doctors avoid ineffective or more costly approaches that might not work or, worse, allow a patient's condition to deteriorate by delaying more effective treatment.

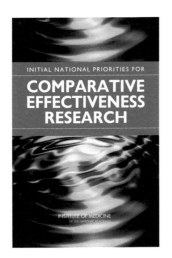

The IOM report, *Initial National Priorities for Comparative Effectiveness Research* (2009), provides 100 top priorities for comparative effectiveness research. These priorities should play into decisions regarding the $400 million appropriated for comparative effectiveness research in the American Recovery and Reinvestment Act.

Embracing health information technologies

The old adage "knowledge is power" may apply especially to health care. Yet many sectors of the health care system have been slow to embrace information technologies. In a recent report, for example, the American Hospital Association found that only 11 percent of hospitals had fully implemented use of electronic health records, while another 57 percent had partially implemented their use. To help foster progress in applying information technology to health care, the HHS in 2004 established the Office of the National Coordinator for Health Information Technology (ONC) and set a 10-year goal for creating the Nationwide Health Information Network. For guidance on its efforts to advance its health agenda, HHS turned to the IOM.

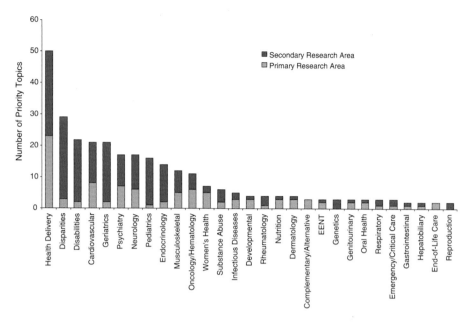

Distribution of the recommended research priorities by primary and secondary research areas.

SOURCE: Initial National Priorities for Comparative Effectiveness Research, p. 101.

The IOM's Board on Health Care Services, in collaboration with the National Research Council's Computer Science and Telecommunications Board, examined the cohesiveness and pace of the HHS program, focusing in particular on efforts to develop and implement operating standards. *Opportunities for Coordination and Clarity to Advance the National Health Information Agenda: A Brief Assessment of the Office of the National Coordinator for Health Information Technology: A Letter Report* (2007) finds a number of shortcomings in current efforts and points to needed improvements.

In sum, the study committee was unable to make a straightforward assessment of the pace of activities, in large part because the ONC had not set forth a clear and complete set of milestones against which such an assessment could be made. The report notes that some observers believe the process (from the selection of use cases to standards acceptance) is proceeding too slowly, while others believe it is going too quickly. These views reflect varying perceptions about the standards processes as a whole as well as concerns about whether a uniform pace is appropriate for all activities.

The report advises the head of the ONC to develop a strategic plan—as required by the Executive Order that established the office—providing a roadmap with specific objectives, milestones, and metrics for the national health information technology agenda. The ONC also should clarify how it will accomplish its aims, focusing specifically on processes for making program decisions, for managing workflow, for coordinating efforts within the program and with other groups, and for obtaining feedback and incorporating it into program operations. These steps can help capitalize on the promise that information technology holds for improving the nation's health.

Exploring the prospects of integrative medicine

At a time when attention has turned to health reform and the future shape of health care, many are considering the promise of "integrative medicine." Integrative medicine can be described as orienting the health care process to engage patients and caregivers in the full range of physical, psychological, social, preventive, and therapeutic factors known to be effective and necessary for the achievement of optimal health.

With support from The Bravewell Collaborative, the IOM convened the Summit on Integrative Medicine and the Health of the Public in February 2009 to explore the science and practice of integrative medicine for improving the breadth and depth of patient-centered care and promoting the nation's health. During the meeting, participants reviewed the state of the science, assessed the potential and the priorities, and began to suggest elements of an agenda to help improve the prospects for integrative medicine's contributions to better health and health care. Speakers and attendees also discussed the ways in which integrative medicine seeks to encourage the personal and community environments that shape and empower patients' knowledge, skills, and support to be active participants in their own care.

Ensuring that those who need care can receive care

The nation's health care system not only must be efficient and deliver high-quality services. The system also must be properly structured and complemented by a range of other government policies in order to ensure that everyone has ready and equal access to health services.

Seeking solutions for the nation's uninsured crisis

The growing number of uninsured Americans—totaling 45.7 million as of 2007—is taking a toll on the nation's health. One in 5 adults under age 65 and nearly 1 in 10 children are uninsured. Uninsured individuals experience much more risk to their health than insured individuals.

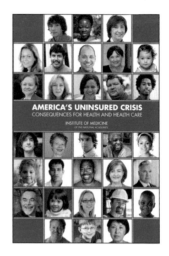

Between 2001 and 2004, the IOM issued six reports on the consequences of being uninsured and offering a uniform recommendation—namely, that the nation quickly implement a strategy to achieve health insurance coverage for all. With support from The Robert Wood Johnson Foundation, the IOM returned to this issue in 2008 and produced an up-to-date assessment of the research evidence regarding insurance coverage. *America's Uninsured Crisis: Consequences for Health and Health Care* (2009) finds that a chasm remains between the health care needs of people without health insurance and access to effective health care services. This gap results in needless illness, suffering, and death.

The evidence shows more clearly than ever that having health insurance is essential for people's health and well-being, and safety-net services are not enough to prevent avoidable illness, worse health outcomes, and premature death. Moreover, new research suggests that when local rates of uninsurance are relatively high, even people with insurance are more likely to have difficulty obtaining needed care and to be less satisfied with the care they receive. Without concerted attention from all stakeholders, these problems will only grow worse as the current economic crisis and associated growth in unemployment fuel further decline in the number of people with health insurance and intensify financial pressures on local health care delivery.

The growing number of uninsured Americans—totaling 45.7 million as of 2007—is taking a toll on the nation's health. One in 5 adults under age 65 and nearly 1 in 10 children are uninsured.

Reducing health disparities and promoting health literacy

For many of those who do have health insurance, proper health care remains a fantasy more than reality. Although the health status for many U.S. resi-

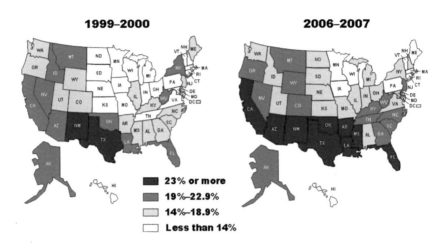

Comparison in the percentage of nonelderly adults without health insurance, by state, 1999–2000 and 2006–2007.

SOURCE: America's Uninsured Crisis: Consequences for Health and Health Care, p. 14.

dents has improved steadily, some racial and ethnic groups—including African Americans, Hispanics, Native Americans, Alaskan Natives, Asians, and Pacific Islanders—find themselves excluded from such progress. Members of these groups more frequently develop diseases such as cancer, HIV infection and AIDS, cardiovascular disease, asthma, stroke, and diabetes, and their infants suffer higher rates of mortality. Across these groups, tens of millions of people experience health levels, as measured in terms of life expectancy, that are more typical of those in developing countries.

The IOM's Roundtable on Health Disparities convened a workshop to increase the visibility of racial and ethnic health disparities as a national problem, further the development of programs and strategies to reduce disparities, and foster leaders who can advance the field. *Challenges and Successes in Reducing Health Disparities: Workshop Summary* (2008) presents the experiences of health professionals and other care workers who serve on the front lines of efforts to reduce disparities in health care, as well as the experiences of researchers, policy makers, community activists, and other individuals who deal with the array of social factors that help determine a person's overall health.

Based on their various experiences, some participants called for increased efforts at the national level to collect solid data about health disparities and eliminate institutional racism. Other participants focused on

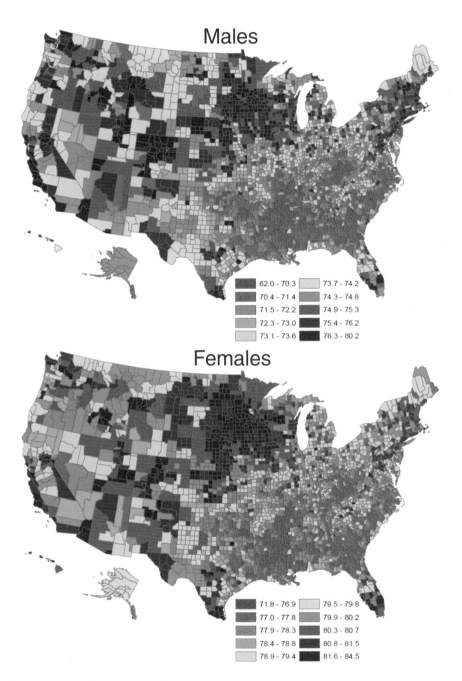

Males

62.0 - 70.3	73.7 - 74.2
70.4 - 71.4	74.3 - 74.8
71.5 - 72.2	74.9 - 75.3
72.3 - 73.0	75.4 - 76.2
73.1 - 73.6	76.3 - 80.2

Females

71.8 - 76.9	79.5 - 79.8
77.0 - 77.8	79.9 - 80.2
77.9 - 78.3	80.3 - 80.7
78.4 - 78.8	80.8 - 81.5
78.9 - 79.4	81.6 - 84.5

County life expectancy 1997–2001.

SOURCE: Challenges and Successes in Reducing Health Disparities: Workshop Summary, p. 9.

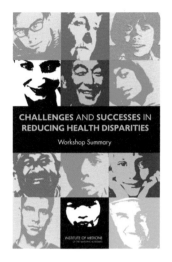

the local level, suggesting, for example, that communities develop the capacity to gather their own health, social, and economic data, rather than rely on standard indicators alone. In this way, communities will be able to track the health status of their members over time, enabling them to call for help from state or national organizations as needed to correct any health problems that emerge.

As the nation has experienced vast demographic changes, especially over the past generation as waves of immigrants dispersed across the country and formed new communities, new challenges have emerged in the way the health care system delivers services. Health care providers now must tailor their efforts to each individual, reflecting that person's culture and languages. The aim is to ensure that all patients receive the same quality of care and that they have adequate knowledge and understanding of health issues and services to make appropriate decisions about their care.

This transformation has incidentally elevated health care disparities and health literacy as major health care topics. Three IOM bodies—the Forum on the Science of Health Care Quality Improvement and Implementation, the Roundtable on Health Disparities, and the Roundtable on Health Literacy—jointly convened a workshop in 2008 to discuss these concerns. *Toward Health Equity and Patient-Centeredness: Integrating Health Literacy, Disparities Reduction, and Quality Improvement: Workshop Summary* (2009) explores the various steps that health professionals and others are taking to improve care delivery to today's populations and what challenges remain in assuring better health for future populations.

Workshop participants, drawn from a range of fields across the health care spectrum, examined how providing patients with appropriate medications in their primary languages and offering translation services can vastly improve the health care patients receive, and they considered ways in which health care providers might integrate these seemingly separate challenges into their daily routines. Participants discussed how providers can best manage available resources and how they can teach health literacy over the life course of their patients. They also considered how improvements at the national level in areas such as data collection and workforce training can positively affect health care and improve health outcomes.

Largest Disparities in Health Care Quality for Selected Groups: 2005 Versus 2007 NHDR[a]

Group	2005 NHDR[a]		2007 NHDR[a]	
	Measure	Relative Rate	Measure	Relative Rate
Black	New AIDS cases per 100,000 population age 13 and over	10.4	New AIDS cases per 100,000 population age 13 and over	10.0
	Hospital admissions for pediatric asthma per 100,000 population ages 2–17	4.0	Hospital admissions for pediatric asthma per 100,000 population ages 2–17	3.8
	Percent of patients who left the emergency department without being seen	1.9	Hospital admissions for lower extremity amputations in patients with diabetes per 100,000 population	3.8
Asian	Persons age 18 or older with serious mental illness who did not receive mental health treatment or counseling in the past year	1.6	Composite: Adults who reported poor communication with health providers	1.6
	Adults who can sometimes or never get care for illness or injury as soon as wanted	1.6	Long-stay nursing home residents who were physically restrained	1.5
	Adults age 65 and over who did not ever receive pneumococcal vaccination	1.5	Adults age 65 and over who did not ever receive pneumococcal vaccination	1.5
AI/AN[b]	Women not receiving prenatal care in the first trimester	2.1	Women not receiving prenatal care in the first trimester	2.1
	Composite: Adults who reported poor communication with health providers	1.8	Composite: Adults who reported poor communication with health providers	1.8

continued

Continued

Group	2005 NHDR[a] Measure	Relative Rate	2007 NHDR[a] Measure	Relative Rate
	Children ages 2–17 with no advice about physical activity	1.3	Women age 40 and over who reported they did not have a mammogram within the past 2 years	1.8
Hispanic	New AIDS cases per 100,000 population age 13 and over	3.7	New AIDS cases per 100,000 population age 13 and over	3.5
	Adults who can sometimes or never get care for illness or injury as soon as wanted	2.0	Hospital admissions for lower- extremity amputations in patients with diabetes per 100,000 population	2.9
	Composite: Children whose parents reported poor communication with their health providers	1.8	Women not receiving prenatal care in the first trimester	2.0
Poor	Composite: Children whose parents reported poor communication with their health providers	3.3	Composite: Children whose parents reported poor communication with their health providers	3.0
	Adults who can sometimes or never get care for illness or injury as soon as wanted	2.3	Adults who can sometimes or never get care for illness or injury as soon as wanted	2.4
	Children ages 2–17 who did not have a dental visit	2.0	Women age 40 and over who reported they did not have a mammogram within the past 2 years	2.1

[a]NHDR = National Healthcare Disparities Report.

[b]AI/AN = American Indian/Alaska Native.

SOURCE: Toward Health Equity and Patient-Centeredness: Integrating Health Literacy, Disparities Reduction, and Quality Improvement: Workshop Summary, p. 10.

Stretching Across International Borders

In spring 2009, a new type of influenza appeared in Mexico and quickly spread to the United States and around the world. Its cause: a mutated strain of swine flu virus—labeled H1N1 influenza A by scientists. Thousands of people fell seriously ill, and though most recovered, some did not.

The outbreak underscores the message that health threats recognize no political or geographic borders. Indeed, given today's increasingly interconnected world, new or reemerging diseases are no more than an airplane ride—or even a car ride—away. Moreover, global events, ranging from climate disruption to poverty and violence, threaten public health as well.

In this era of globalization, the United States has a key role to play in maintaining health and mitigating risk. The Institute of Medicine (IOM) examines different aspects of this responsibility. The IOM looks at how the nation can best protect its own residents from global health threats and also at how the nation can help other countries with limited resources to tackle health problems within their own borders.

Meeting the global need for U.S. commitment

In 2008, the IOM—with the support of four federal agencies and five private foundations—formed an independent committee to examine the nation's current and future role in global health. The committee issued a report in two installments, the first specifically targeting recommendations to government and the second offering recommendations for the public and private sectors as well. The report as a whole revisits the IOM's 1997 study *America's Vital Interest in Global Health*, which argued that a firm commitment by the United States to promote health around the world serves not only the international population, but also the American people.

The U.S. Commitment to Global Health: Recommendations for the New Administration (2008), the first installment of the new report, calls for highlighting health as a pillar of U.S. foreign policy and backing this up with significant funding increases for global health efforts over the next 4 years. It lays out a broad path for how the President and administration can demonstrate their commitment to global health:

- Expanding and rebalancing the federal government's aid portfolio, particularly by increasing funding for chronic, noncommunicable diseases, which account for more than half of all deaths in low- and middle-income countries.

- Creating a White House Interagency Committee on Global Health, composed of heads of major federal departments and agencies involved in global health, and designating a senior administration official as its leader.

- Improving evaluation in order to determine which interventions are working and which are not.

- Developing and implementing an expanded research agenda— supporting, in particular, new research targeting health problems specific to poor populations—that could yield new tools, such as a vaccine for malaria, for use in global health programs.

- Ensuring that health improvements will be sustainable by working with pivotal international groups, such as the World Health Organization; partnering with other national governments; and strengthening local health systems and workforces.

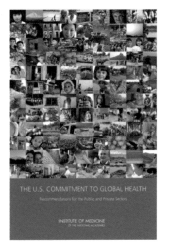

The U.S. Commitment to Global Health: Recommendations for the Public and Private Sectors (2009), the second installment, provides a more detailed action plan that requires the participation of every sector of the U.S. global health enterprise. It calls on U.S.-based commercial entities, foundations, universities, and other nonprofit organizations to join with the government in taking action in five key areas:

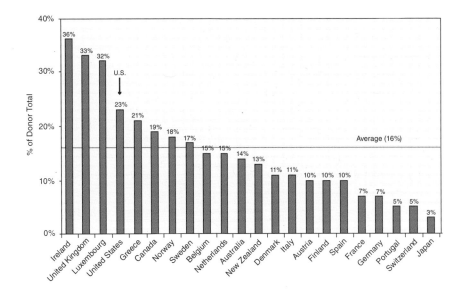

Allocable aid for health (2006).

SOURCE: The U.S. Commitment to Global Health: Recommendations for the Public and Private Sectors, p. 134.

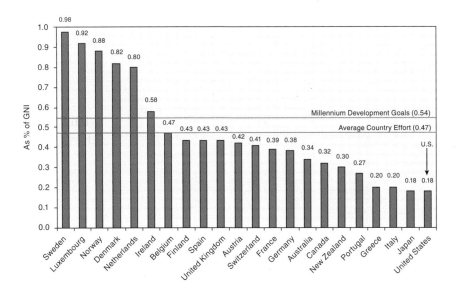

Net official development assistance (2008).

SOURCE: The U.S. Commitment to Global Health: Recommendations for the Public and Private Sectors, p. 135.

1. Scaling up proven interventions for improving health outcomes and reducing poverty, a known contributor to health problems, in low- and middle-income countries. Numerous interventions are available, but many nations lack the infrastructure or resources to take sufficient action on their own.

2. Generating and sharing knowledge that serves the global community. Typically, the United States and other wealthy countries focus their health research on conditions that affect their own people. This situation too often means that the tools to prevent and treat many diseases in resource-limited countries are either inadequate or not fully used because there is insufficient understanding of how best to apply them in such settings.

3. Investing in capacity building with global partners. Many countries face critical health workforce deficits that directly affect efforts at combating disease and death. U.S. institutions should establish long-term partnerships with universities, research centers, and health care systems in resource-limited countries to help them build a cadre of capable local leaders and researchers who can identify effective solutions to health problems that are sustainable in their own countries.

4. Increasing financial commitments to global health. Although the U.S. government has made record commitments to global health, its overall commitment to overseas development assistance falls below the efforts of other developed countries. The government also should consider novel approaches, such as results-based financing, to delivering aid that is effective.

5. Setting an example by engaging in respectful partnerships. To ensure that countries retain ownership and accountability for the health of their people, the United States should support resource-limited countries in developing results-focused, country-led agreements that rally all development partners around one health plan, one monitoring and evaluation framework, and one review process.

International aid focusing on global health is a longstanding tradition in the United States, and the White House increased its commitments under President George W. Bush. On July 30, 2008, President Bush signed into law a reauthorization of the President's Emergency Plan for AIDS Relief (PEPFAR), originally launched in 2003, providing $15 billion in relief. The new law expanded funding more than threefold, to $48 billion, to treat not only AIDS, but also tuberculosis and malaria. The reauthorization eliminated a previous requirement that one-third of all prevention funding must go to abstinence and fidelity programs, as well as other earmarks to allow local implementers to allocate funds based on the needs of at-risk populations. These modifications, along with an increased focus placed on women and girls, were recommended in the 2007 IOM report *PEPFAR Implementation: Progress and Promise*, a congressionally mandated evaluation of the program.

Yet the reach of global health goes far beyond worldwide disease prevention and international relations. It is an interdisciplinary field that also incorporates economics, epidemiology, and public health, among others. One area that tends to be overlooked is violence, which may include interpersonal and self-directed violence, violence in society, violence in the family, and violence against women and children, among others. Such violence, comprising both suicidal behavior and interpersonal violence, is among the leading causes of death and disability worldwide. In 2000 alone, the latest year for data, violence claimed an estimated 1.6 million lives globally—more than 1.5 times the number of deaths from malaria. The devastating impact of violence also extends far beyond immediate death, resulting in injuries that are often lifelong, hospitalizations, political instability, and stagnation of economic growth for families, communities, and nations. Although it strikes everywhere, violence overwhelmingly and disproportionately affects low- and middle-income countries, which often lack the resources to invest in prevention and to respond to the consequences of violence.

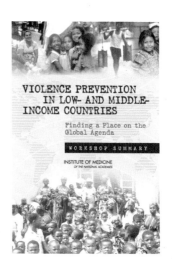

The IOM, together with the nonprofit group Global Violence Prevention Advocacy, convened a workshop to examine how a public health approach might be applied in lessening the pressing dangers. Among their goals, workshop participants—drawn from an array of fields related to health, criminal justice, public policy, and economic development—set out to discuss specific opportunities for the U.S. government and other public and private groups with resources to more effectively support programs aimed at preventing the many forms of violence that occur. *Violence Prevention in Low- and Middle-Income Countries: Finding a Place on the Global Agenda: Workshop*

Summary (2008) highlights the need for the timely development of an integrated, science-based agenda to support research, clinical practice, program development, policy analysis, and advocacy for violence prevention.

In 2000 alone, the latest year for data, violence claimed an estimated 1.6 million lives globally—more than 1.5 times the number of deaths from malaria.

One central message is that the current state of science in violence prevention reveals progress, promise, and a number of remaining challenges. Most of what is known about effective violence prevention comes from studies in developed countries, but improved collaboration could help developing countries apply these lessons to their own circumstances. Promising, effective interventions are currently being implemented in and by developing countries, but they have not been rigorously evaluated for scaling up to regional and national levels. Both government and private efforts are needed to span this knowledge gap.

Top 10 Causes of Death, Ages 5-44 Years, Both Sexes, 2002

Rank	5-14 Years	15-29 Years	30-44 Years
1	Childhood cluster 200,139	HIV/AIDS 855,406	HIV/AIDS 855,406
2	Road traffic injuries 118,212	Road traffic injuries 354,692	Tuberculosis 368,501
3	Drowning 113,614	Tuberculosis 238,021	Road traffic injuries 354,692
4	Respiratory infections 112,739	Self-inflicted injuries *216,661*	Ischemic heart disease 224,986
5	Diarrheal diseases 88,430	Interpersonal violence *188,451*	Self-inflicted injuries *215,263*
6	Malaria 76,257	War injuries *95,015*	Interpersonal violence *146,751*
7	HIV/AIDS 46,022	Drowning 78,639	Cerebrovascular disease 145,965
8	War injuries *43,671*	Respiratory infections 65,153	Cirrhosis of the liver 135,072
9	Tuberculosis 36,362	Poisonings 61,865	Respiratory infections 102,431
10	Tropical diseases 31,845	Fires 61,341	Liver cancer 84,279

NOTE: Bold, italic figures highlight deaths or disability due to violence.

SOURCE: Violence Prevention in Low- and Middle-Income Countries: Finding a Place on the Global Agenda: Workshop Summary, p. 25.

Confronting infectious diseases

In recent decades, most of the emerging infectious disease events in humans have been caused by zoonotic pathogens—those infectious agents that are transmitted from animals to humans. Noteworthy changes in the patterns of human and animal contact in recent years make conditions ripe for global outbreaks of zoonotic diseases, the 2009 swine flu outbreak among them. Some of these diseases, including AIDS, severe acute respiratory syndrome (SARS), and West Nile virus infection, have already caused global health and economic crises. With an estimated billion people crossing international borders every year, the shipment of animals and animal products over great distances to reach their final destinations, and rampant population growth in countries where poverty rates are high and people by necessity live in close proximity to animals, new outbreaks could emerge with devastating health, economic, environmental, agricultural, and sociopolitical results.

The IOM and the National Research Council jointly convened a workshop to examine how well the United States and the world are prepared to deal with the threats of zoonotic diseases over the long term. *Achieving Sustainable Global Capacity for Surveillance and Response to Emerging Diseases of Zoonotic Origin: Workshop Summary* (2008) outlines what is known about the transmission of zoonotic disease and explores the current global capacity for zoonotic disease surveillance. In particular, the report discusses methods of disease surveillance as a way of detecting outbreaks of diseases in animals, spotting outbreaks of zoonotic disease in humans, and using these data to inform public health responses to outbreaks or perhaps prevent them in the future. It also describes components of a research plan to explore many of the questions that remain about how best to protect humans worldwide from the transfer and spread of diseases from animals.

Changing climatic conditions also have contributed to a shift in the global spread of disease. Climatic change has long been known to influence the appearance and spread of epidemic diseases, but evidence is mounting that Earth's climate is changing at a faster rate than previously appreciated and that this change likely will be accompanied by more frequent occurrences of extreme weather events, such as droughts and hurricanes. This awareness is leading researchers to view the relationships between climate and disease with a new urgency and from a global perspective.

The IOM explored various aspects of this climate–health link at a workshop convened by its Forum on Microbial Threats. *Global Climate*

Change and Extreme Weather Events: Understanding the Contributions to Infectious Disease Emergence: Workshop Summary (2008) notes that the projected impacts of climate change and extreme weather events are pre-

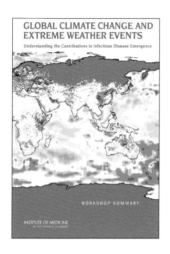

dominately negative. Impacts are expected to be most severe in low-income countries where the capacity to adapt is weakest, though developed countries also are vulnerable, as was demonstrated in 2003 when tens of thousands of Europeans died as a result of record-setting summer heat waves.

The report discusses some of the scientific questions that must be answered in order to discern—and, ultimately, to predict—the effects of a changing climate on specific infectious diseases, as well as to identify technical means to tackle these issues. For example, it will be critical to develop a greater understanding of the interaction of climate with other major factors, such as the globalization of travel and trade, population growth, urbanization, land-use patterns, and habitat destruction, that play a role in disease emergence and resurgence. Governments also will need to establish long-term monitoring programs to simultaneously track climate and infectious disease dynamics, and to optimize measurement instruments (many of which were designed for other purposes) for use in such programs. In addition, researchers must continue to develop and refine predictive models of climate and infectious disease as the basis for early warning and public health response systems, and governments should encourage more stakeholders to become involved in the operation of such systems.

Assessing treatment of disease

Malaria is a leading cause of death among children in the developing world. Of the more than 1 million people who die of malaria each year, more than 80 percent are young children in sub-Saharan Africa. One promising approach for reducing malaria's toll is called intermittent preventive treatment, in which all infants, regardless of whether or not they are infected, are given a full therapeutic course of an antimalarial drug—typically sulfadoxine-pyrimethamine—at defined intervals, usually in conjunction with regularly scheduled visits to health clinics. But questions have remained about the method's effectiveness.

Observed Changes in North American Extreme Events, Assessment of Human Influence for the Observed Changes, and Likelihood That the Changes Will Continue Through the Twenty-first Century[a]

Phenomenon and Direction of Change	Where and When These Changes Occurred in Past 50 Years	Linkage of Human Activity to Observed Changes	Likelihood of Continued Future Changes in This Century
Warmer and fewer cold days and nights	Over most land areas, the last 10 years had lower numbers of severe cold snaps than any other 10-year period	Likely warmer extreme cold days and nights and fewer frosts[b]	Very likely[d]
Hotter and more frequent hot days and nights	Over most of North America	Likely for warmer nights[b]	Very likely[d]
More frequent heat waves and warm spells	Over most land areas, most pronounced over northwestern two-thirds of North America	Likely for certain aspects, e.g., night-time temperatures; and linkage to record high annual temperature[b]	Very likely[d]
More frequent and intense heavy downpours and higher proportion of total rainfall in heavy precipitation events	Over many areas	Linked indirectly through increased water vapor, a critical factor for heavy precipitation events[c]	Very likely[d]
Increases in area affected by drought	No overall average change for North America, but regional changes are evident	Likely, Southwest USA.[c] Evidence that 1930s and 1950s droughts were linked to natural patterns of sea surface temperature variability	Likely in Southwest USA, parts of Mexico, and Carribean[d]

continued

Continued

Phenomenon and Direction of Change	Where and When These Changes Occurred in Past 50 Years	Linkage of Human Activity to Observed Changes	Likelihood of Continued Future Changes in This Century
More intense hurricanes	Substantial increase in Atlantic since 1970; likely increase in Atlantic since 1950s; increasing tendency in W. Pacific and decreasing tendency in E. Pacific (Mexico West Coast) since 1980[e]	Linked indirectly through increasing sea surface temperature, a critical factor for intense hurricanes;[e] a confident assessment requires further study[c]	Likely[d]

[a]Based on frequently used family of Intergovernmental Panel on Climate Change emission scenarios.

[b]Based on formal attribution studies and expert judgment.

[c]Based on expert judgment.

[d]Based on model projections and expert judgment.

[e]As measured by the Power Dissipation Index (which combines storm intensity, duration, and frequency).

SOURCE: Global Climate Change and Extreme Weather Events: Understanding the Contributions to Infectious Disease Emergence, p. 7.

At the request of the Bill & Melinda Gates Foundation, which is investing heavily in malaria treatment and prevention worldwide, the IOM convened an expert committee to examine the body of evidence about the technique's effectiveness. The committee relied heavily on work conducted by the Intermittent Preventive Treatment in Infants Consortium, comprising 17 leading organizations involved in malaria research in Africa, Europe, and the United States. *Assessment of the Role of Intermittent Preventive Treatment for Malaria in Infants: Letter Report* (2008) concludes that the method yields significant benefits. Some reported data, for example, showed that treated infants experienced approximately 20 to 30 percent fewer clinical malaria episodes than did untreated infants.

Based on such findings, the report concludes that intermittent preventive treatment is worthy of further investment as part of a public health strategy to decrease morbidity from malaria infections among infants who are at high risk because they reside in malaria-endemic areas. The report also recommends, however, that if public health authorities elect to expand use of the method in sub-Saharan Africa, they should include monitoring efforts during the early stages to further assess their safety, effectiveness, cost effectiveness, acceptability, and sustainability at the community level.

Because malaria kills so many people and is an enormous public health problem, health experts around the world are searching for new ways to fight the disease. While the recent IOM report discusses intermittent preventive treatment, that is only one option among many. In 2004, the IOM released *Saving Lives, Buying Time: The Economics of Antimalarial Drugs*, which recommended ways to make the new combination malaria treatments—called artemisinin-combination therapies, or ACTs—widely accessible despite their high cost. The report's central recommendation came to pass in April 2009 with the announcement of a program called Affordable Medicines Facility for Malaria. Funded by international public health organizations and European governments, the program will be piloted in Cambodia and 10 African countries initially, and then evaluated after 2 years to determine its success and viability.

Although it may not claim as many lives each year as malaria, influenza poses an even broader geographic sweep of health challenges. During the early stages of an influenza pandemic, physicians and other public health workers may rely on two antiviral drugs, oseltamivir (sold as Tamiflu®) and zanamivir (sold as Relenza®), to treat illness and slow its spread during the several months it takes to develop a vaccine. But as the emergence of a new strain of flu virus in spring 2009 demonstrated, it is difficult to estimate in advance how severe the next pandemic will be and what mix of treatment and prophylaxis will be optimal.

At the request of the U.S. Department of Health and Human Services (HHS), the IOM examined the nation's strategies for coping with major new influenza outbreaks. *Antivirals for Pandemic Influenza: Guidance on Developing a Distribution and Dispensing Program* (2008) concludes that governments at all levels—federal, state, and local—currently lack a coordinated plan to get drugs fairly and efficiently to people who need them. The report calls for government officials to begin a national and public process of creating an ethical framework for allocating antivirals, and for the federal government to appoint a science-based advisory body that can guide decision making during a pandemic.

Prioritized Strategies for Antiviral Drug Use from November 2007 HHS Draft Proposed Guidance

Population to Receive Prophylaxis	Estimated Number of Antiviral Courses Needed
Initial pandemic outbreaks overseas and in the United States	6 million
Exposed travelers entering the United States early in a pandemic	
Persons with pandemic influenza illness (outbreak and post-exposure)	79 million
Health care and emergency services workers	103 million
Outbreak control in closed settings (e.g., nursing homes)	5 million
Immunocompromised and not candidates for vaccine	2 million
Unique and specialized infrastructure workers	2 million
Household contacts of cases *The summary of the proposed guidance, dated November 20, 2008, revises the preliminary position on household prophylaxis: "No national recommendation is made at this time for PEP [post-exposure prophylaxis] of household contacts of an influenza case or for workers in sectors other than healthcare and emergency services."*	*88 million*
Total estimated number of courses for treatment and prophylaxis	285 million
Total excluding household post-exposure prophylaxis	*197 million*

SOURCE: Antivirals for Pandemic Influenza: Guidance on Developing a Distribution and Dispensing Program, p. 29.

In developing a strategic framework, officials should establish, among other things, a process for prioritizing which groups of people should first receive antiviral medications currently stored in federal and state stockpiles. In most instances, first priority should go to health care workers and emergency personnel who are likely to face repeated viral exposures, followed by other health care providers and emergency responders, and then people in households in which a member has been infected. The prioritization process should be built to have enough flexibility to adjust for the particular circumstances of an actual outbreak, including how quickly the virus spreads, which population groups it affects most severely, and how readily it responds to drugs.

In addition to engaging the public in prioritization planning, government officials also should connect with the corporations and other private entities that are building stockpiles of antiviral drugs for their employees. Efforts to establish agreements and understanding between the public and private sectors could lead to collaboration in an actual outbreak and reduce confusion and inefficiencies during a pandemic.

In most instances, first priority should go to health care workers and emergency personnel who are likely to face repeated viral exposures, followed by other health care providers and emergency responders, and then people in households in which a member has been infected.

While malaria and influenza remain everyday threats to human health, in the late 20th century the global health community eradicated one of the most devastating diseases ever to plague humanity: smallpox. Today, all known stocks of the disease's causative agent, variola virus, are stored in two repositories sanctioned by the World Health Organization—in the United States at the federal Centers for Disease Control and Prevention, and in Russia at the State Centre for Research on Virology and Biotechnology. But debate has continued about whether to retain or destroy these stocks of live virus.

In 1999, the Institute of Medicine explored this question, and its report, *Assessment of Future Scientific Needs for Live Variola Virus*, concluded that preserving live strains of the virus could help researchers in developing medical countermeasures for smallpox. That same year, the World Health Assembly, the decision-making body of the World Health Organization, declared that given the important research remaining, a decision about retaining stocks of the live virus should be deferred until 2010.

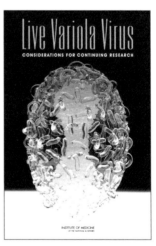

To help prepare for this decision, the HHS and the Centers for Disease Control and Prevention requested the IOM review the body of research that has accumulated over the past decade and determine what unmet needs still exist that require the use of live variola virus. *Live Variola Virus:*

Overview of Essential Versus Useful Scientific Needs for Live Variola Virus

Need	Requires Use of Live Virus	Does Not Require Live Virus
Essential	• Development of therapeutics and assessment of resistance • Development of vaccines that do not manifest a take	• Development of first- and second-generation vaccines that produce a take • Development of methods for detection and diagnosis
Useful	• Functional genomics–based research • Discovery research	• Variola genome sequence analysis

SOURCE: Live Variola Virus: Considerations for Continuing Research, p. 4.

Considerations for Continuing Research (2009) finds that developing medical countermeasures against this deadly pathogen remains an essential need because of the potential for an accidental or deliberate release, and that having access to stocks of live variola virus will critically aid researchers in reaching their goals. The report singles out four areas for particular attention: development of improved therapeutics; development of new or improved vaccines; genomic analysis to improve the fundamental understanding of the virus and identify new strategies for therapies; and "discovery research" that can yield fundamental insights about human biology as well as lessons on how to improve smallpox prevention and treatment.

Eating Right:
Keeping America Healthy

A healthy nation is a well-nourished nation, in which all people eat enough of what they need to and avoid, as much as possible, foods that are not healthful. For the United States, this remains an ideal. The nation has made progress toward this goal, but falls short in a number of areas and even has slipped backward in some instances.

The Institute of Medicine (IOM) has a long history of examining the nation's nutritional well-being—where things stand, what is going right, what needs to be done. Two key areas have received particular attention: improving nutrition among children and adolescents, who are developing rapidly and thus are especially sensitive to nutritional shortcomings, and coming to grips with the epidemic of obesity that is spreading among many sectors of the population.

Educating children and teens

Students in southwestern Kentucky are proving to be wily innovators in improving their own health, through a program sponsored by the IOM and the Healthy Weight Kids Coalition in Kentucky, and their efforts may chart a way for other young people to take charge of their eating habits. The program traces back to an IOM project in 2006 during which students in a number of middle and high schools in and around Bowling Green, Kentucky, gathered information about the food and beverage marketing practices in their region. In thinking about how healthful foods might be marketed better, particularly toward youth, one student suggested providing incentives to use "healthy smart cards"—magnetized cards approved specifically for purchasing healthful food items—when eating at local restaurants.

The idea caught hold. Through its Kellogg Health of the Public Fund and in partnership with the Healthy Weight Kids Coalition and Western Kentucky University, the IOM began a new effort to explore the potential of healthy smart cards in helping young people make better food choices. Program coordinators identified food options at local restaurants, recruited restaurants to participate in the program, developed educational and promotional materials, and procured community support. They developed the cards that students could use, designed and distributed point-of-purchase displays and other materials for restaurants, installed card readers and trained workers on how to use them, and looked for ways to encourage student participation. After learning from students that a website would be helpful in educating students about the program and also hosting other program resources, the team developed both a paper guidebook and a website to help youth identify the healthy options available at various local restaurants.

Ten restaurants (including McDonald's and Chick-fil-A franchises) committed to displaying information about the program, installing card readers, and offering discounts on healthful food purchases when students presented their cards. Supporters lined up, including most city and county schools, local hospital systems and health care providers, the local restaurant association, and the city's mayor.

The Smart Bites Card Program, as it is called, rolled out in January 2009 with great fanfare, with more than 50 percent of the eligible students signing up to participate. Over the long term, the IOM hopes the program will prove to be replicable across the United States.

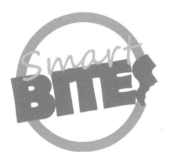

In addition to educating young people about healthful foods, the nation also must find ways to ensure that children have the opportunity to make healthy choices. The IOM has tackled this issue through many recent activities: the establishment of a new committee to help guide the IOM's work on obesity prevention; an evaluation of the national school meal program and assessment of how it might be updated; and hosting a workshop to discuss "food deserts"—low-income neighborhoods with limited access to affordable, nutritious food; in addition to other nascent studies.

Fighting fat

Despite progress over the past century in improving the health of the nation's children, recent years have seen a new threat emerge and spread—an epidemic of childhood obesity. It is occurring in boys and girls in all 50 states, in younger children as well as adolescents, across all socioeconomic strata, and among all ethnic groups—though specific subgroups, including African Americans, Hispanics, and American Indians, are disproportionately affected. Nationwide, approximately 9 million children over the age of 6 are considered obese, and health professionals and policy makers now rank childhood obesity as a critical public health threat.

Nationwide, approximately 9 million children over the age of 6 are considered obese, and health professionals and policy makers now rank childhood obesity as a critical public health threat.

To help in slowing, and ultimately reversing, this epidemic, the IOM has examined childhood obesity on numerous occasions. For example, *Preventing Childhood Obesity: Health in the Balance* (2005) played a landmark role documenting the severity of the problem and the complexity of and need for many sectors to work together to find solutions. *Food Marketing to Children and Youth: Threat or Opportunity?* (2006) offered recommendations for different segments of society—government, schools, families, food and restaurant industries, and the media, among others—to guide the development of effective marketing and advertising strategies that promote more healthful foods, beverages, and meal options. *Nutrition Standards for Foods in Schools: Leading the Way Toward Healthier Youth* (2007) outlines nutritional standards for the availability, sale, content, and consumption of foods at school. The standards are designed to promote consumption of fruits, vegetables, whole grains, and nonfat or low-fat dairy products and limit the consumption of saturated fat, salt, added sugars, caffeine, and total calories. The IOM's report *Progress in Preventing Childhood Obesity: How Do We Measure Up?* (2007) took stock of progress since 2005 and found that while innovative and encouraging actions were happening across the United States, many efforts are fragmented and small in scale. The report's recommenda-

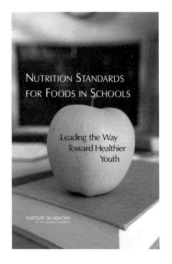

tions emphasize the need for a collective responsibility and collaborative actions among all who have a stake in reversing the epidemic, and it provides a framework to evaluate how projects are working.

To build on this foundation, the IOM established the Standing Committee on Childhood Obesity Prevention in 2008, with support from The Robert Wood Johnson Foundation. Bringing together experts representing a range of fields and drawn from government, academia, and the corporate sector, the committee serves as a focal point for national and state-level discussions. By convening workshops in targeted areas and helping to select topics for study by outside independent committees, the aim is to foster effective, comprehensive, and coordinated efforts to combat this growing problem.

A Framework for Decision Making for Obesity Prevention: Integrating Action with Evidence was generated in collaboration with the standing committee. This report, expected in spring 2010, will determine a framework for policy makers and community leaders to make decisions about obesity prevention, specifically how they might affect food, eating, and physical activity environments.

Reviewing national school meal programs

Improving the school lunch and breakfast programs can have a direct impact on the health of youth. Tens of millions of students nationwide receive as much as half of their daily caloric intake from school meals, including breakfasts and lunches, provided through federal programs. For children in families facing limited resources, school meals provide a critical safety net.

Tens of millions of students nationwide receive as much as half of their daily caloric intake from school meals, including breakfasts and lunches, provided through federal programs.

Yet the programs' meal requirements and nutrition standards have gone unchanged for more than a decade, making them out of step with recent guidance about the nutritional needs of children and adolescents. Early on, the programs focused primarily on overcoming nutrient deficiencies and underconsumption. But as many overt deficiencies in children's diets largely have been eliminated, other nutrition-related concerns have emerged, most notably a high prevalence of childhood obesity.

At the request of the U.S. Department of Agriculture, which administers the meals programs, the IOM is evaluating the programs and will recommend updates to improve their performance. The recommendations are intended to reflect new developments in nutrition science and to increase the availability of key food groups offered in the programs. The study committee will work in two phases, the first of which was completed in 2008. *Nutrition Standards and Meal Requirements for National School Lunch and Breakfast Programs: Phase I. Proposed Approach for Recommending Revisions* (2008) provides an overview of the school meal programs and their participants, reviews what is known about children's food and nutrient needs and deficiencies, and describes the committee's proposed planning model and analytic methods for developing its recommendations. The second report,

Foods and Nutrients Under Consideration in Children's Diets

Age Category	Foods for Which Intakes Are Inadequate, Male and Female	Nutrients for Which Intakes Are Inadequate		Nutrients for Which Intakes Are Excessive[a]	
		Male	Female	Male	Female
Ages 6–8[b]	Fruit Total vegetables Dark green and orange vegetables and legumes Whole grains Total meat and beans Milk	Potassium Fiber	Potassium Fiber	Sodium Saturated fat Total fat Energy[c]	Sodium Saturated fat Total fat Energy[c]
Age 9–13	Fruit Total vegetables Dark green and orange vegetables and legumes Whole grains Total meat and beans Milk	Magnesium Potassium Vitamins A, E Fiber	Calcium Magnesium Phosphorus Potassium Zinc Vitamins A, C, E Fiber	Sodium Cholesterol Saturated fat	Sodium Energy[c] Total fat Saturated fat

continued

Continued

Age Category	Foods for Which Intakes Are Inadequate, Male and Female	Nutrients for Which Intakes Are Inadequate		Nutrients for Which Intakes Are Excessive[a]	
		Male	Female	Male	Female
Age 14–18	Fruit Total vegetables Dark green and orange vegetables and legumes Whole grains Total meat and beans Milk	Magnesium Potassium Vitamins A, C, E Energy[c] Fiber	Calcium Iron Magnesium Phosphorus Potassium Zinc Vitamins A, C, E, B_6, B_{12} Folate Thiamin Energy[c] Fiber	Sodium Cholesterol Saturated fat Total fat	Sodium Cholesterol Saturated fat Total fat

NOTE: Excessive energy intakes for some age-gender groups may not have been identified because of underreporting.

[a] Excessive amounts of discretionary calories were consumed from solid fat and added sugars; this also constitutes concern relative to recommendations to be made by the committee. Usual intakes of added sugars could not be estimated because relevant data were not available in School Nutrition Dietary Assessment Study-III. Furthermore, while intakes of *trans* fatty acids also could not be measured, *trans* fatty acids will be considered as appropriate by the committee during Phase II.

[b] Data for children age 5 years were included in the food intake data.

[c] It is difficult to accurately estimate energy intakes because of under- and overreporting of food intake and a lack of accurate information about customary levels of physical activity.

SOURCE: Nutrition Standards and Meal Requirements for National School Lunch and Breakfast Programs: Phase I. Proposed Approach for Recommending Revisions, p. 10.

which is expected in fall 2009, will specify the updated nutrition standards and meal standards.

Determining nutrient needs

For consumers to make the best choices about what they eat, they need sound information about food and nutrition. The National Academies has been providing such information for nearly seven decades. The IOM's Food and Nutrition Board has issued more than three dozen sets of guidelines— first called Recommended Daily Allowances and recently replaced and expanded as Dietary Reference Intakes (DRIs). Developed by U.S. and Canadian scientists, the DRIs provide quantitative estimates of the amounts of nutrients that individuals need to optimize their health and prevent disease and deficiencies, as well as estimates of tolerable upper intake levels to help people avoid adverse effects from consuming too much of a nutrient. DRIs are widely used by a range of health professionals and policy makers, including federal nutrition officials who develop policies and programs, dietitians and health practitioners who counsel individuals and groups, and researchers who are working to advance the state of nutrition knowledge.

The IOM convened a workshop in 2007—attended by research scientists, nutrition practitioners, government officials from the United States and Canada, and industry representatives, among others—to survey a decade-long slice of this experience. *The Development of DRIs 1994–2004: Lessons Learned and New Challenges: Workshop Summary* (2008) explores a variety of issues that emerged during this period and outlines how past experience can help guide decisions about the next phase in developing DRIs and putting them to work in promoting the public's health.

New and relevant research on vitamin D and calcium has prompted the U.S. and Canadian governments to request a review of DRIs for vitamin D and calcium. The work is under way and a report is expected in spring 2010.

Managing Threats and Ensuring Healthy Communities: Health of the Public

Public health is fundamental to every individual's health. An Institute of Medicine (IOM) committee in 1988 described the mission of public health as fulfilling society's interest in assuring conditions in which people can be healthy. Yet each individual's health and well-being are shaped by the interactions of genetic endowment, environmental exposures, lifestyle and food choices, social conditions, income, and medical care. Collectively, these factors shape health at the population level—the domain of public health.

As a reflection of its broad spectrum, public health is perhaps the most diverse area the IOM investigates.

As a reflection of its broad spectrum, public health is perhaps the most diverse area the IOM investigates. The studies deal with important—and sometimes contentious—challenges that affect people from every walk of life, in every part of the country.

Preventing disease, early detection, and effective treatment

Since its founding, the IOM has consistently stressed the value of prevention of disease, a core tenet of public health. In studies ranging from core principles and needs in the field to specific issues such as health disparities, vaccine safety, smoking cessation, and reducing environmental hazards, the IOM continues to advance the best ways to ensure the public's health.

Improving vaccines

In the United States and worldwide, vaccines have proved to be the most potent and cost-effective means of controlling infectious diseases. However, vaccines have yet to achieve their full potential.

In 1994, the U.S. government implemented a National Vaccine Plan that charted a route to more fully capture the promise of vaccines. Administered by the National Vaccine Program Office (NVPO) of the Department of Health and Human Services, the plan had four main goals: to develop new and improved vaccines; to ensure the optimal safety and effectiveness of vaccines and immunization; to better educate the public and members of the health professions on the benefits and risks of immunizations; and to achieve better use of existing vaccines to prevent disease, disability, and death. The plan, which offered more than 70 strategies for achieving its objectives, has recorded numerous successes since its implementation. But recent years also have kindled awareness that the plan needs to be modified to meet new challenges and opportunities.

Working in coordination with a number of federal agencies, the NVPO now is in the preliminary stages of updating the plan, and the partners turned to the IOM for assistance. *Initial Guidance for an Update of the National Vaccine Plan: A Letter Report to the National Vaccine Program Office* (2008) examines the goals, objectives, strategies, and anticipated outcomes of the original plan; explores how it was developed; and critiques the initial draft update that was proposed. Based on this analysis, the report identifies six specific "content" areas in which technical aspects of the 1994 plan might be improved and four "methodology" areas that might be strengthened in the process of updating the plan.

The report urges the inclusion of stakeholders beyond federal agencies in framing the plan's scope, goals, and objectives. Additional contributors should include the pharmaceutical industry, insurers, health care providers and other purchasers of health care services, researchers across a range of basic and applied sciences, state and local public health agencies responsible for vaccine delivery, schools and day care centers, foundations and other not-for-profit organizations, the mass media, and, importantly, the public (including people with varying perspectives on the value of immunization), among others. Following the release of this initial guidance, the committee began its review of the draft update of the vaccine plan, which will be released late in 2009. It convened meetings of stakeholders in medicine, public health, and vaccinology to discuss the five goals laid out in the draft plan.

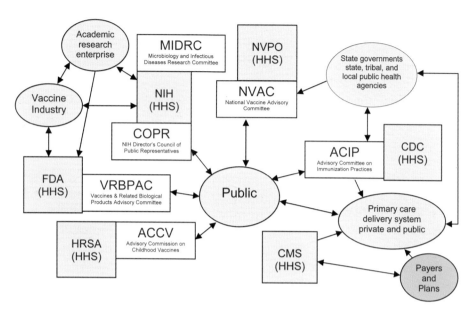

FIGURE 6-1 Federal advisory committees and Department of Health and Human Services (HHS) agencies associated with vaccine- or immunization-specific programs.

NOTE: This figure is intended to illustrate some aspects of the immunization system's complexity, not to be a complete description of the system. A number of federal advisory committees exist to provide advice and guidance to agencies in HHS. Four such committees, as well as two additional relevant committees, are depicted in the figure.

Legend: Gray boxes represent federal agencies in HHS (other departments, such as the Departments of Defense, Veterans Affairs, and Homeland Security, also play important roles in the immunization system); white boxes represent federal advisory committees associated with HHS agencies, and gray ovals represent other stakeholders.

Acronyms: CDC = Centers for Disease Control and Prevention; CMS = Centers for Medicare & Medicaid Services; FDA = Food and Drug Administration; HRSA = Health Resources and Services Administration; NIH = National Institutes of Health; NVPO = National Vaccine Program Office.

ACCV includes attorneys for injured children and for industry; NVAC Includes public, industry, state public health, and health care (AHIP) representation; ACIP includes public and state and local public health representation and liaisons to the vaccine industry and professional associations; COPR includes patients, family members of patients, health care and education professionals and members of the general public who advise the Director of the NIH on "matters of public interest, outreach and participation in NIH's research-related activities;" VRBPAC includes public and nonvoting industry representation.

SOURCE: Initial Guidance for an Update of the National Vaccine Plan: A Letter Report to the National Vaccine Program Office, p. 9.

For many years the IOM has been involved in evaluating evidence concerning adverse health effects that may be associated with specific vaccines covered by the Vaccine Injury Compensation Program. In 2009, the IOM began a new study to review the epidemiological, clinical, and biological evidence relating to the health effects of varicella zoster vaccine, influenza vaccines, hepatitis B vaccine, human papillomavirus vaccine, and possibly others. The upcoming reports will consider whether a specific vaccine is related to a specific adverse event.

Helping to improve medication safety

Each year, people taking medications as outpatients experience more than a million harmful consequences that result in a trip to a physician's office or an emergency room. Sometimes, such adverse reactions lead to hospitalization or even death. A patient's first line of defense against medication hazards is the label on the drug's container that provides information about the drug and how it should be taken. Yet research shows that nearly half of all patients have trouble understanding label instructions, either because of some type of literacy limitation or because the labels are poorly presented.

. . . research shows that nearly half of all patients have trouble understanding label instructions, either because of some type of literacy limitation or because the labels are poorly presented.

The IOM's Roundtable on Health Literacy examined this safety issue in a workshop that brought together a diverse array of participants, including representatives from government, the pharmacy field, the health care community, the research enterprise, and the public, among others. *Standardizing Medication Labels: Confusing Patients Less: Workshop Summary* (2008) surveys what is known about how medication container labeling affects patient safety and describes participants' various suggestions for fixing the problem.

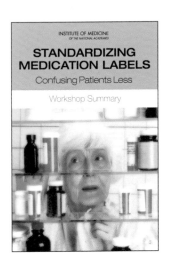

Many patients do not understand current drug labels, but the best way to improve comprehension of medication instructions is unclear. Experts differ in their judgments about exactly what information should be included on a drug label and how that information should be presented. Although there have been some tests of various types of labels, workshop participants concluded that more research is needed to find answers that are both broader and more precise. There is also disagreement about whether regulation or a voluntary approach will best achieve label standardization, with some participants

Patient Misunderstanding of Medication Instructions

Dosage Instruction	Patient Interpretation
Take one teaspoonful by mouth three times daily	Take three teaspoons daily Take three tablespoons every day Drink it three times a day
Take one tablet by mouth twice daily for 7 days	Take two pills a day Take it for 7 days Take one every day for a week I'd take a pill every day for a week
Take two tablets by mouth twice daily	Take it every 8 hours Take it every day Take one every 12 hours

SOURCE: Standardizing Medication Labels: Confusing Patients Less: Workshop Summary, p. 15.

favoring each approach and arguing that the other has not been proven successful.

In providing a possible way forward, the report offers a list of questions for an expanded research program. What are the mechanisms by which standardization can be achieved? What would the process look like? What are the costs of standardizing? What level of evidence is needed to introduce a best practice? At the same time, care must be taken to ensure that steps to promote label standards do not detract from other efforts, such as education of both patients and physicians in matters of drug safety, that are needed to reduce medication errors.

Reducing environmental and foodborne threats

Many public health concerns stem from some type of agent that humans release into the environment. This release may result from the activities of society—for example, from industries that emit chemical pollutants—or from the actions of individuals, as in the instance of cigarette smoking. In either case, the public has an interest in better understanding and eliminating all such hazards.

Reviewing Great Lakes pollution studies

The Great Lakes are magnificent—and environmentally critical—resources for both the United States and Canada. But many sections of the lakes are contaminated with a variety of potentially hazardous pollutants. In 1972, the two nations signed the Great Lakes Water Quality Agreement to restore and maintain the lakes' chemical, physical, and biological integrity. Under the agreement, the International Joint Commission monitors and assesses the nations' activities, including efforts to protect human health from contaminants. In 2001, the commission asked the Agency for Toxic Substances and Disease Registry (ATSDR), part of the U.S. Centers for Disease Control and Prevention (CDC), to evaluate the public health implications of hazardous materials present in U.S. portions of the lakes. (The commission also has worked with Health Canada to document conditions in Canadian waters.)

After a first unsuccessful attempt, the ATSDR produced a draft report in 2007. Even then, registry officials had concerns about the methods used and the conclusions drawn in the draft, and the registry released a revised draft report in 2008. This further revision attracted criticism of its scientific integrity, however, and the CDC asked the IOM to conduct an independent study. *Review of the ATSDR's Great Lakes Report Drafts: Letter Report* (2008) concludes that both drafts have shortcomings that diminish

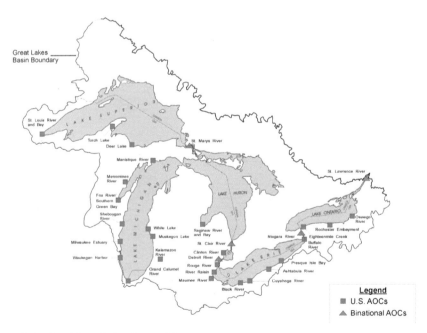

U.S. and Binational Great Lakes Areas of Concern.

NOTE: AOCs = Areas of Concern.

SOURCE: Review of the ATSDR's Great Lakes Report Drafts: Letter Report, p. 33.

their scientific quality and limit their usefulness in determining whether health risks might be associated with living near the lakes. The report item- izes a number of faults—often involving data selection—and explains their adverse consequences. Many of the problems appear to stem from the lack of a clear statement of objectives and an approach to reach those aims.

The report suggests ways to approach similar tasks in the future. Such projects should begin by identifying the research questions to be answered or the tasks to be undertaken, and then should develop and document a detailed approach to answering those research questions. The group under- taking the project also should seek out other entities for partnering, such as federal agencies or state governments, as early in the process as possible.

Improving food safety

In support of strengthening the U.S. food safety system, IOM worked with the Division of Earth and Life Studies to help the U.S. Department of Agri- culture to improve its risk-based inspection system. Additionally, a con- gressionally mandated review of the Food and Drug Administration's role in ensuring safe food is underway and will be completed by summer 2010.

Improving emergency preparedness

In today's world, the United States must be prepared to respond to a vari- ety of hazards, both natural events and deliberate actions taken by other nations or terrorist groups. Ensuring a high degree of preparedness remains a never-ending concern. The IOM recognizes that preparing for emergen- cies and disasters is crucial to protecting the public's health. The organiza- tion has devoted many resources to helping federal agencies prepare for national emergencies that may arise, with particular focus during the past few years on emerging diseases.

In 2008–2009, the IOM held a workshop on the capacity of the health care system to treat an affected population in the case of a nuclear event; published a report discussing how the global health community can strengthen surveillance and response to emerging zoonotic diseases; and will release late in the year another report that evaluates the Department of Homeland Security's BioWatch program, which is intended to detect airborne biological threats. Three previous IOM reports provide insights into how government might respond to an outbreak of pandemic influenza

Key Elements of Preparedness

A prepared community is one that develops, maintains, and uses a realistic preparedness plan that is integrated with routine practices and has the following components:

Preplanned and coordinated rapid-response capability

1. *Health risk assessment*. Identify the hazards and vulnerabilities (e.g., community health assessment, populations at risk, high-hazard industries, physical structures of importance) that will form the basis of planning.

2. *Legal climate*. Identify and address issues concerning legal authority and liability barriers to effectively monitor, prevent, or respond to a public health emergency.

3. *Roles and responsibilities*. Clearly define, assign, and test responsibilities in all sectors, at all levels of government, and with all individuals, and ensure each group's integration.

4. *Incident Command System (ICS)*. Develop, test, and improve decision making and response capability using an integrated ICS at all response levels.

5. *Public engagement*. Educate, engage, and mobilize the public to be full and active participants in public health emergency preparedness.

6. *Epidemiology functions*. Maintain and improve the systems to monitor, detect, and investigate potential hazards, particularly those that are environmental, radiological, toxic, or infectious.

7. *Laboratory functions*. Maintain and improve the systems to test for potential hazards, particularly those that are environmental, radiological, toxic, or infectious.

8. *Countermeasures and mitigation strategies*. Develop, test, and improve community mitigation strategies (e.g., isolation and quarantine, social distancing) and countermeasure distribution strategies when appropriate.

9. *Mass health care*. Develop, test, and improve the capability to provide mass health-care services.

10. *Public information and communication*. Develop, practice, and improve the capability to rapidly provide accurate and credible information to the public in culturally appropriate ways.

11. *Robust supply chain*. Identify critical resources for public health emergency response and practice and improve the ability to deliver these resources throughout the supply chain.

Expert and fully staffed workforce

1. *Operations-ready workers and volunteers*. Develop and maintain a public health and health-care workforce that has the skills and capabilities to perform optimally in a public health emergency.

2. *Leadership*. Train, recruit, and develop public health leaders (e.g., to mobilize resources, engage the community, develop interagency relationships, and communicate with the public).

Accountability and quality improvement

1. *Testing operational capabilities*. Practice, review, report on, and improve public health emergency preparedness by regularly using real public health events, supplemented with drills and exercises when appropriate.

2. *Performance management*. Implement a performance management and accountability system.

3. *Financial tracking*. Develop, test, and improve charge capture,[a] accounting, and other financial systems to track resources and ensure adequate and timely reimbursement.

[a]Charge capture systems collect and analyze charges for medical care.

SOURCE: Research Priorities in Emergency Preparedness and Response for Public Health Systems: A Letter Report, p. 11.

or other infectious disease threats. These reports speak to the use of face masks and other personal protective equipment in health care settings. All emphasize the vital importance of meeting the needs of the health care workers and other front-line personnel who provide care for others during an influenza pandemic.

As part of a national effort to ensure security, Congress in 2006 enacted the Pandemic and All Hazards Preparedness Act, which called for refocusing the research priorities of the network of Centers for Public Health Preparedness now operating at 27 accredited schools of public health nationwide. The federal government had created the centers in 1999 to provide expanded expertise to strengthen the nation's emergency response systems, and the new law both refined and expanded that charge.

To help with this restructuring, the agency that oversees the centers, the Coordinating Office for Terrorism Preparedness and Emergency Response (COTPER), which is part of the CDC, asked the IOM to develop a research agenda that can be carried out over the next 3 to 5 years. *Research Priorities in Emergency Preparedness and Response for Public Health Systems: A Letter Report* (2008) proposes that the centers give priority to four general areas. These include research (1) to design and implement emergency preparedness training and for translating the results into public use, (2) to communicate accurate information in a timely manner to diverse audiences, (3) to create sustainable community-based preparedness systems, and (4) to generate improved criteria and metrics for evaluating the performance of public health emergency response systems.

Less than a month after the IOM released its report, COTPER issued a request for applications for research grants that incorporated almost verbatim the report's findings and recommendations. COTPER expects to award nearly $9 million to projects that "investigate the structure, capabilities, and performance of public health systems for preparedness and emergency response activities."

Taking Care of Those Who Take Care of Us: Military and Veterans

The men and women in the United States armed forces confront health challenges of a scope and complexity that few other Americans ever experience. Active-duty personnel in combat directly face risks of injury or death. In addition, both combat forces and personnel serving away from the front lines may experience lengthy exposures to hazardous environments, either natural or produced by human activities. Chemical exposures, for example, may at times exceed those that would be considered safe in a civilian working environment. Beyond immediate physical threats, military personnel often must deal with the effects of being in high-intensity, stressful, and dangerous environments, sometimes for months or years at a time.

The Department of Defense (DoD) bears the primary responsibility for keeping troops fit for service, protecting service men and women from preventable risks, and providing them with high-quality health care. The Department of Veterans Affairs (VA) provides health care to service members after they leave the military. In order to help fulfill these missions, the DoD and the VA regularly turn to the Institute of Medicine (IOM) to study and recommend actions on a range of health-related issues.

Assessing the health effects of the Gulf War

In 1991, nearly 700,000 U.S. troops, including many members of the reserve and National Guard, took part in the Persian Gulf War. On returning home, a substantial number of military personnel reported health problems that they believed to be connected to their service. At the request of Congress, the IOM has conducted a series of studies that examine the scientific and medical evidence on the health effects of the various agents to which military personnel may have been exposed during the Gulf War. The IOM more recently expanded its focus to include studies on the health effects experienced by military personnel involved in the war in Afghanistan, which began in 2001, and the war in Iraq, which began in 2003.

The IOM published the first volume in the *Gulf War and Health* series in 2000. It assesses the health effects of exposure to a variety of chemicals, including depleted uranium and the warfare agent sarin, as well as the health effects that may be related to use of pyridostigmine bromide and vaccines, including the botulinum toxoid and anthrax vaccines. (An update to this report, focused specifically on sarin, was released in 2004.) The second volume in the series, published in 2003, examines the health effects associated with exposure to pesticides and solvents. The third volume, published in 2005, analyzes the long-term human health effects associated with exposure to selected environmental agents, pollutants, and other synthetic chemical compounds, such as fuels and propellants. The fourth volume, published in 2006, examines the state of veterans' health in the years since the conflict, rather than specific potential causes of health problems. The fifth volume, published in 2007, examines the long-term health effects associated with various infectious diseases that Gulf War veterans—as well as veterans of the Afghanistan and Iraq wars—may have faced.

Evaluating the effects of combat stress

The sixth volume in the series focuses on health effects linked to the stresses of serving in a combat zone. By definition, war zones are stressful places. Troops face concerns about surviving, being taken prisoner, or being tortured. They may see friends die or become maimed, and they may have to handle dead bodies. Less traumatic but more pervasive stressors include anxiety about home life, such as loss of a job and income, impacts on relationships, and absence from family.

Gulf War and Health, Volume 6: Physiologic, Psychologic, and Psychosocial Effects of Deployment-Related Stress (2007) finds that military personnel who serve in war zones face a greater risk of developing posttraumatic stress disorder (PTSD), other anxiety disorders, and depression than do personnel who are not deployed. They also are more likely to experience alcohol abuse, accidental death, suicide, and marital and family conflict, including domestic violence, within the first few years after leaving the war zone. In addition, drug abuse, unexplained illnesses, chronic fatigue syndrome, gastrointestinal symptoms, skin diseases, fibromyalgia, chronic pain, and an increased likelihood of being incarcerated may be associated with the stresses of being in a war, although the evidence to support these links is weaker. The findings are based not only on studies of Gulf War veterans, but also on studies of veterans from World War II, the Korean War, the Vietnam War, and the wars in Afghanistan and Iraq.

The report notes that it is not yet possible to offer definitive answers about the connections between many health problems and the stresses of war, in part because the military does not routinely assess service members' physical, mental, and emotional status before deployment. This knowledge gap is taking on increased importance as the United States continues its military operations in Iraq and expands them in Afghanistan. To help bridge the gap, the DoD should conduct comprehensive, standardized evaluations of service members' medical conditions, psychiatric symptoms and diagnoses, and psychosocial status and trauma history before and after they deploy to war zones. Such screenings would provide baseline data for comparisons and information to determine the long-term consequences of deployment-related stress. In addition, they would help identify at-risk personnel who might benefit from targeted intervention programs, such as marital counseling or therapy for psychiatric or other disorders, during deployment, and they would help the DoD and the VA choose which intervention programs to implement for veterans adjusting to postdeployment life. A separate IOM study, described later in this chapter, specifically discusses treatment of PTSD.

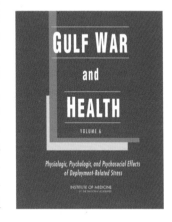

Evaluating the effects of brain injury

War is damaging in any form, but the wars in Afghanistan and Iraq have brought new types of weaponry and methods of attack that have proved increasingly dangerous. In particular, these conflicts are seeing expanded use of more powerful explosive devices that are causing more severe types of blast injuries, especially traumatic brain injury. Indeed, traumatic brain

Summary of Findings Regarding the Association Between Deployment to a War Zone and Specific Health and Psychosocial Effects

Sufficient Evidence of a Causal Association
Evidence from available studies is sufficient to conclude that there is a causal relationship between deployment to a war zone and a specific health outcome in humans. The evidence is supported by experimental data and fulfills the guidelines for sufficient evidence of an association (below). The evidence must be biologically plausible and satisfy several of the guidelines used to assess causality, such as strength of association, dose-response relationship, consistency of association, and temporal relationship.
- No effects.

Sufficient Evidence of an Association
Evidence from available studies is sufficient to conclude that there is a positive association. That is, a consistent positive association has been observed between deployment to a war zone and a specific health outcome in human studies in which chance and bias, including confounding, could be ruled out with reasonable confidence. For example, several high-quality studies report consistent positive associations, and the studies are sufficiently free of bias and include adequate control for confounding.
- Psychiatric disorders, including PTSD, other anxiety disorders, and depressive disorders.
- Alcohol abuse.
- Accidental death in the early years after deployment.
- Suicide in the early years after deployment.
- Marital and family conflict.

Limited but Suggestive Evidence of an Association
Evidence from available studies is suggestive of an association between deployment to a war zone and a specific health outcome, but the body of evidence is limited by the inability to rule out chance and bias, including confounding, with confidence. For example, at least one high-quality study reports a positive association that is

sufficiently free of bias, including adequate control for confounding, and other corroborating studies provide support for the association (corroborating studies might not be sufficiently free of bias, including confounding). Alternatively, several studies of lower quality show consistent positive associations, and the results are probably not due to bias, including confounding.

- Drug abuse.
- Chronic fatigue syndrome.
- Gastrointestinal symptoms consistent with functional gastro-intestinal disorders, such as irritable bowel syndrome or functional dyspepsia.
- Skin disorders.
- Fibromyalgia and chronic widespread pain.
- Increased symptom reporting, unexplained illness, and chronic pain.
- Incarceration.

Inadequate/Insufficient Evidence to Determine Whether an Association Exists

Evidence from available studies is of insufficient quantity, quality, or consistency to permit a conclusion regarding the existence of an association between deployment to a war zone and a specific health outcome in humans.

- Cancer.
- Diabetes mellitus.
- Thyroid disease.
- Neurocognitive and neurobehavioral effects.
- Sleep disorders or objective measures of sleep disturbance.
- Hypertension.
- Coronary heart disease.
- Chronic respiratory effects.
- Structural gastrointestinal diseases.
- Reproductive effects.
- Homelessness.
- Adverse employment outcomes.

continued

Continued

Limited/Suggestive Evidence of No Association

Evidence from well-conducted studies is consistent in not showing a positive association between exposure to a specific agent and a specific health effect after exposure of any magnitude. A conclusion of no association is inevitably limited to the conditions, magnitudes of exposure, and length of observation in the available studies. The possibility of a very small increase in risk after exposure studied cannot be excluded.

  • No effects.

SOURCE: Gulf War and Health, Volume 6: Physiologic, Psychologic, and Psychosocial Effects of Deployment-Related Stress, p. 8.

injury has come to be the signature wound of the war in Iraq, with more than 5,500 soldiers suffering such injury as of early 2008.

Gulf War and Health, Volume 7: Long-Term Consequences of Traumatic Brain Injury (2008) finds that military personnel who suffer moderate or severe degrees of such injuries face an increased risk for developing several health problems at some time in their lives. These problems include symptoms similar to Alzheimer's and Parkinson's diseases, aggression, memory loss and impaired concentration, depression, and diminished abilities to maintain social relationships. Some personnel who suffer even mild traumatic brain injury also experience some of these health consequences, including increased risk for aggressive behavior, depression, and memory and concentration problems. Traumatic brain injury may cause other adverse consequences as well, such as vision problems and seizures, a particular type of diabetes, psychosis, and suicide, though there is not sufficient evidence to make definitive conclusions.

... traumatic brain injury has come to be the signature wound of the war in Iraq, with more than 5,500 soldiers suffering such injury as of early 2008.

The report emphasizes the need to develop a fuller picture of the effects of traumatic brain injuries and other blast injuries. Toward this end,

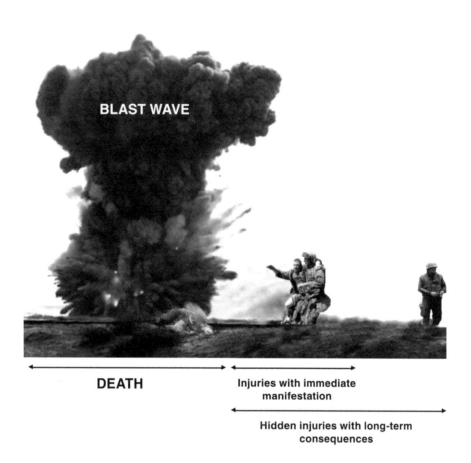

Potential consequences of blast exposure.

SOURCE: Gulf War and Health, Volume 7: Long-Term Consequences of Traumatic Brain Injury, p. 30.

the DoD should make use of several available diagnostic and evaluative tools to study every soldier who has a history of blast exposure, even of low intensity. It also should conduct predeployment neurocognitive tests of all military personnel to establish a baseline for identifying postinjury consequences, and it should conduct postdeployment neurocognitive testing of representative samples of military personnel, including those who have and have not suffered traumatic brain injury. In addition, the VA should include uninjured service members and other comparison groups in the Traumatic Brain Injury Veterans Health Registry that the agency is developing.

The DoD and the VA also should work with the broader research community to develop new or improved clinical and animal testing methods to answer an array of questions. One area of interest, for example, centers on determining the long-term effects of brain injuries sustained as a result of exposure to the force of an explosion without a direct strike to the head—one of the most common perils for soldiers in Iraq and Afghanistan. Problems stemming from such injuries currently may be underdiagnosed, and wounded service members may be losing valuable time for therapy and rehabilitation.

Congress has begun to take note. Shortly after the report's release, Senator Patty Murray (D-WA), a senior member of the Senate Committee on Veterans' Affairs, issued a statement calling for increased screening and research related to traumatic brain injury and declaring her intention to work with the Obama administration "to implement the recommendations outlined by the Institute of Medicine."

In other follow-on activities, the IOM and the National Academy of Engineering convened a workshop to discuss potential tools and techniques for improving the care of patients with traumatic brain injury. Participants, including both engineering and health experts, considered ways to better design care practices for service members treated at multiple institutions within the military, the VA, and the civilian sector.

Evaluating the health effects of depleted uranium

The Gulf War marked the first time that the U.S. military made extensive use of depleted uranium, using it to strengthen tank armor and to increase the penetrating ability of tank munitions. The military continues to use depleted uranium for such purposes in the Iraq war. Depleted uranium is a by-product of the uranium enrichment process used to generate fuel for nuclear power plants. It is abundant and inexpensive, and its chemical and physical properties give it added strength and a high melting point—valuable traits for military use. However, although depleted uranium is less potent than natural uranium, it still emits a significant amount of radiation, and the IOM has conducted several recent studies to better understand the risks that military personnel may face from such exposure.

In 2000, when the IOM issued its initial report on depleted uranium and various other chemical agents, few studies of health outcomes of such exposure had been conducted. The report concluded that there was inadequate or insufficient evidence to determine whether an association exists between uranium exposure and 14 types of adverse health outcomes that were considered possible. Since then, however, the results of additional studies have become available, including studies specifically on exposure to depleted uranium, and the VA asked the IOM to update its review.

Gulf War and Health: Updated Literature Review of Depleted Uranium (2008) finds that the evidence is still inadequate or insufficient to determine whether an association exists between exposure to depleted uranium and all of the health outcomes examined. This list includes lung cancer, leukemia, lymphoma, bone cancer, renal cancer, bladder cancer, brain cancer, stomach cancer, prostate cancer, testicular cancer, reproductive or developmental dysfunction, nonmalignant respiratory disease, gastrointestinal disease, and immune-mediated disease, among others.

Given the many remaining health unknowns, the IOM, at the request of Congress, also explored how epidemiologic studies of veterans might best be conducted to determine the health effects of exposure to depleted uranium on soldiers and on any of their children born after their exposure. Soldiers may be exposed to depleted uranium through a variety of means, including being close to tanks that are attacked and burned, participating in clean-up and salvage operations, or being caught in friendly fire incidents, among others. During the Gulf War, an estimated 134 to 164 people experienced high levels of exposure to depleted uranium, and hundreds or thousands more may have experienced lower exposure through inhalation of contaminated dust particles or ingestion via hand-to-mouth contact with contaminated clothing or other items.

During the Gulf War, an estimated 134 to 164 people experienced high levels of exposure to depleted uranium, and hundreds or thousands more may have experienced lower exposure through inhalation of contaminated dust particles or ingestion via hand-to-mouth contact with contaminated clothing or other items.

Epidemiologic Studies of Veterans Exposed to Depleted Uranium: Feasibility and Design Issues (2008) concludes that it would be difficult to carry out a comprehensive study with currently available data. Rather, the best option would be to conduct a prospective cohort study if future military operations involve exposure of large numbers of service members to depleted uranium. To detect a statistically significant increase in risk of developing lung cancer, a relatively common cancer, such a study may require following more than 1 million people who become exposed. The success of such studies also will depend on the DoD's ability to collect accurate and complete individual-level exposure information on military personnel who enter a war theater in which depleted-uranium munitions

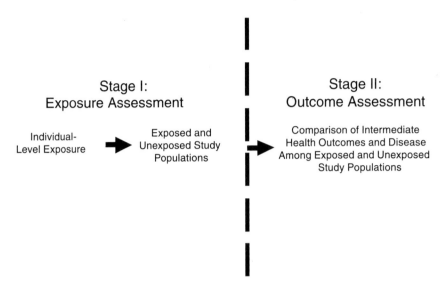

Stages of an epidemiologic study of depleted uranium exposure.

SOURCE: Epidemiologic Studies of Veterans Exposed to Depleted Uranium: Feasibility and Design Issues, p. 7.

and armor are used. In addition, while preparing to conduct such studies, the DoD should work with the research community to advance animal tests and other laboratory methods that may help in expanding the current knowledge base.

Tracking the health effects of Agent Orange

From 1962 to 1971, the U.S. military sprayed herbicides, including a compound called Agent Orange, over Vietnam to strip the thick jungle canopy that could conceal opposition forces, to destroy crops that those forces might depend on, and to clear tall grasses and bushes from the perimeters of U.S. base camps and outlying fire-support bases. Following the war, many veterans and their families began attributing various chronic and life-threatening diseases to exposure to Agent Orange or to dioxin (a contaminant found in the mixture), and in 1991 Congress directed the IOM to study the claims. *Veterans and Agent Orange: Health Effects of Herbicides Used in Vietnam* (1994) provided the first comprehensive, unbiased review of the scientific evidence regarding links between such exposure and various adverse health effects, including cancer, reproductive and developmental problems, and neurobiological disorders. Since then, the IOM has published a series of biennial updates. Collectively, these reports provide the scientific basis on which the VA awards disability compensation to Vietnam veterans. The reports also recommend research that could provide more definitive conclusions about possible health effects.

Even as the IOM carried out its series of studies, one key factor that helps determine health risk remained poorly understood—that is, comprehensive information was lacking about the levels of Agent Orange and other herbicides to which military personnel serving in Vietnam were exposed. To fill this need, a group of academic researchers developed a computer model that characterizes soldiers' exposure based on their proximity to herbicide spraying. Put simply, the model links data on where the military sprayed herbicides with information about troop locations, and then uses the "proximity-based" data to calculate troop exposure levels. But questions have remained about the model's accuracy and reliability, and the VA asked the IOM to analyze the model in order to determine its value, strengths, and limitations.

The Utility of Proximity-Based Herbicide Exposure Assessment in Epidemiological Studies of Vietnam Veterans (2008) finds that, in general, the model offers a promising way to extend knowledge about the effects of herbicides on the health of veterans. The model has certain shortcomings, as does the overall proximity-based approach as a surrogate for determining exposure levels. But the improved ability that the model offers in classifying herbicide exposure, and the application of that information to studies of veterans' health, has value because of its potential to enhance understanding of the health experience of this population.

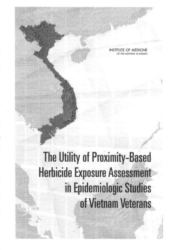

The Utility of Proximity-Based Herbicide Exposure Assessment in Epidemiologic Studies of Vietnam Veterans

The report recommends conducting studies using the model, but it also identifies challenges in applying it and additional research that may strengthen it. For example, conducting epidemiologic studies using the exposure assessment model requires data on when and where each veteran served in Vietnam and on the veteran's health outcomes. But the processes involved in obtaining data on individuals' unit assignments and unit locations are administratively difficult, time consuming, and costly, and the report calls on the VA to work with the DoD and the National Archives and Records Administration to facilitate use of military records in future studies. Even as such studies proceed, however, the VA and other federal agencies should ensure that they be accompanied by other research efforts—including the exploration of other possible exposure models—aimed at reducing the scientific uncertainty about the health of Vietnam veterans.

Fostering the well-being of military personnel

As part of its charge, the U.S. military must protect the health and well-being of its personnel—and their families—in ways that extend beyond bearing arms.

Assessing dietary supplements

Members of the military, like civilians, increasingly are using dietary supplements. Although some supplements may provide benefits to health, others may compromise the readiness and performance of service members. The risks may be greatest for specific military populations, such as members of Special Forces units, who often endure harder tasks and harsher environments and therefore face heightened physiological demands.

The military does not have integrated service-wide policies to guide service members or their commanders on how to use dietary supplements safely. To fill this gap, the DoD and several other public agencies and private groups turned to the IOM. *Use of Dietary Supplements by Military Personnel* (2008) recommends that the military adopt a systematic approach that encompasses three primary strategies: developing a system for monitoring the use of dietary supplements by military personnel, charting a framework for determining which dietary supplements pose the greatest potential problems, and devising a system that soldiers and others and can use to report adverse events associated with dietary supplements. The report also encourages the DoD to appoint an oversight committee or organization to oversee these activities and ensure their performance.

> **The military does not have integrated service-wide policies to guide service members or their commanders on how to use dietary supplements safely.**

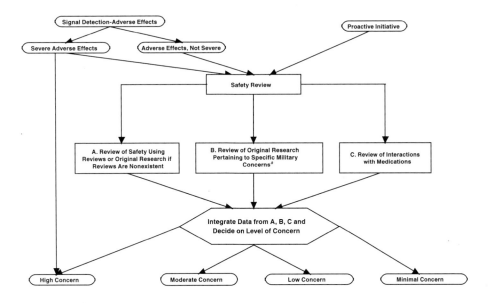

Framework to review the safety of dietary supplements.

[a]High physical activity, calorie restriction, hydration, gastrointestinal tract (diarrhea/nausea), liver health/function (xenobiotic clearance), cardiovascular health, mood/behavior altering, alertness/drowsiness, extreme heat/cold, injury/bleeding.

SOURCE: Use of Dietary Supplements by Military Personnel, p. 7.

In implementing this approach, several activities will be key. Information gathering and sharing must be improved. The various military services should, among other things, continue their periodic surveys, but also conduct additional surveys at selected military bases about dietary supplement use among service members who might face heightened health risks due to their tasks or environment. The services also should increase their educational and outreach efforts to provide soldiers and their families, unit commanders, and health care personnel with accurate, up-to-date information about the effects of dietary supplements and the importance of reporting any adverse effects that result from their use.

Reducing tobacco use

Fewer than 20 percent of Americans use tobacco, but more than 30 percent of active-duty military personnel do. Tobacco use not only endangers individual health, but among military populations, it impairs readiness by reducing physical fitness, visual acuity, and sometimes hearing. Adding to concerns, the increased incidence of tobacco use among service members carries over into civilian life, with about 22 percent of veterans using tobacco.

The DoD and the armed services have set goals and taken some actions to become tobacco free, and the VA has a long history of attempting to reduce smoking among veterans. But problems remain, and the DoD and the VA asked the IOM to review their efforts and recommend improvements. *Combating Tobacco Use in Military and Veteran Populations* (2009) recommends that the DoD and the VA increase the priority they place on reducing tobacco use and back up this commitment by implementing state-of-the-art programs to achieve tobacco-free military and veteran populations. These programs should be run according to a strategic plan with an established time line, enforced by an engaged leadership, supported by adequate resources, and implemented by effective and enforceable policies.

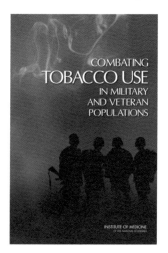

As one key guideline, the report says that achieving a tobacco-free military begins by limiting the number of new tobacco users entering the military and by promoting cessation programs to ensure abstinence. Using a phased approach, the military academies and officer training programs in both universities and the military should become tobacco free first, followed by newly enlisted recruits, and finally by all other active-duty personnel. As an important part of this effort, Congress should change its policy that requires the military to sell tobacco products at reduced prices in its commissaries and exchanges, with the ultimate goal being to prohibit tobacco sales entirely at these outlets. Congress also should repeal its requirement that the VA provide designated smoking areas at its health care facilities, as such provisions have precluded the VA from going entirely tobacco free.

Fewer than 20 percent of Americans use tobacco, but more than 30 percent of active-duty military personnel do.

Identifying the best ways to treat posttraumatic stress disorder

Posttraumatic stress disorder (PTSD) is the most commonly diagnosed service-related mental disorder among military personnel returning from Iraq

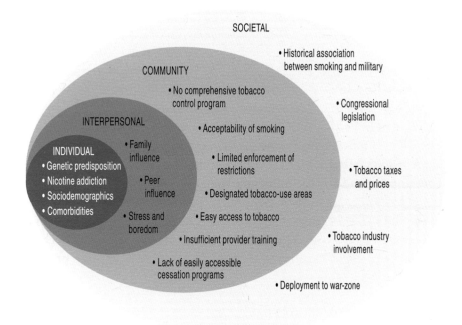

Some of the socioecologic influences on tobacco use among the military and veteran populations.

SOURCE: Combating Tobacco Use in Military and Veteran Populations, p. 82.

and Afghanistan. Surveys indicate that an estimated 12.6 percent of those who fought in Iraq and 6.2 percent of those who fought in Afghanistan have experienced PTSD. Significant numbers of Vietnam veterans and veterans of earlier conflicts also report suffering from PTSD.

Although clinicians now use several drug regimens and psychotherapeutic interventions to treat PTSD, the effectiveness of these therapies remains in question. Many observers suggest that the bulk of the studies have significant scientific shortcomings, and as a result they do not provide a clear picture of what does and does not work. At the request of the VA, the IOM reviewed the literature in an attempt to bring matters into better focus and to identity needed actions.

Treatment of PTSD: An Assessment of the Evidence (2007) concludes that because of shortcomings in many of the studies, there is not enough reliable evidence to draw conclusions about the effectiveness of most treatments. However, there is sufficient evidence to conclude that exposure therapies, such as exposing individuals to a real or surrogate threat in a safe environment to help them overcome their fears, are effective. This finding is not meant to suggest that only exposure therapies should be used to treat PTSD and that other treatments should be discontinued. Rather, the review underscores the urgent need for additional high-quality studies that can assist clinicians in providing the best possible care to veterans and others who suffer from this serious disorder. The report offers a series of recommendations that the VA and others can use to build an effective research program. It also calls on Congress to ensure that the VA and other federal agencies have adequate resources to fund quality research on treatment of PTSD and that all stakeholders—including veterans—are represented in research planning.

> Surveys indicate that an estimated 12.6 percent of those who fought in Iraq and 6.2 percent of those who fought in Afghanistan have experienced PTSD.

Evaluating military medical ethics

Military health professionals play a key role in ensuring the welfare of the service members—and, in some cases, the nonmilitary detainees—they treat. But these professionals sometimes may face ethical conflicts that arise from their responsibilities to their patients and their duties as military officers integrally involved in military operations.

To examine these ethical challenges and explore ways to meet such conflicts and gain optimal results, the IOM held a workshop that brought together stakeholders from a variety of fields, including the military, the health care community, universities, and human rights groups. The workshop proceeded from the premise that military ethical conflicts are best brought to light and discussed by military and civilian leaders rather than relegated to individuals to cope with them alone in situations of stress. To hone discussions, workshop participants focused on two particular instances in which ethical conflicts may arise: when a health professional must make a decision about returning to duty a soldier who has experienced a closed head injury, and when a professional must decide how to handle captured detainees who choose to engage in a hunger strike or other ethically charged activities.

Military Medical Ethics: Issues Regarding Dual Loyalties: Workshop Summary (2008) identifies a number of areas of common ground, but also a number of areas in need of continued discussions. Participants discussed at length the need for transparency in policies and processes related to mili-

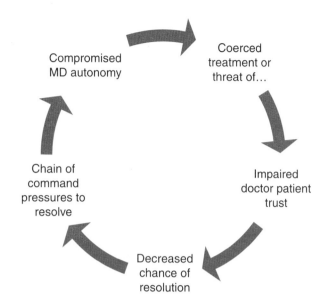

Potential for a spiral of impaired trust in prisons.

SOURCE: Military Medical Ethics: Issues Regarding Dual Loyalties: Workshop Summary, p. 20.

tary ethics, and on the need to seek a wide range of public and professional perspectives when dealing with such issues. They also discussed a need for improvements in training in medical ethics and outlined steps that public and private organizations might take in supporting better ethical awareness and expanded use of ethical standards.

Advancing Knowledge and Shaping a Research Agenda

Situated outside of government and with a broad view of the research enterprise, the Institute of Medicine (IOM) is ideally placed to help guide medical and scientific research and identify priorities for the nation. Government agencies and public organizations alike depend on the findings and recommendations in IOM reports to determine how to structure their ongoing research activities or to embark on new directions. The IOM also looks farther forward to identify opportunities and challenges that lie on— or just over—the scientific horizon.

Examining today's research

Two of today's pressing health concerns illustrate the diversity of challenges in health research and health policy. One centers on the need to find better ways to reduce, and ultimately reverse, the pandemic caused by the human immunodeficiency virus (HIV). The other stems from the accelerating push to electronic medical recordkeeping and its attendant privacy concerns.

Protecting patient privacy while enhancing research

The modern electronic world offers many benefits for health care and health research. Using electronic methods for gathering, sharing, and analyzing patient health information can drive medical advances, including the development of new therapies, improved diagnostics, and more effective ways to prevent illness and deliver care. But the free flow of information also creates the need for privacy protections to ensure that health care and research are carried out in ways that preserve patients' dignity and protect them from harms such as discrimination or identity theft.

In 1996, Congress enacted the Health Insurance Portability and Accountability Act (HIPAA), which called for a set of federal standards, now known as the HIPAA Privacy Rule, for protecting the privacy of personally identifiable health information. Since then, some privacy advocates, researchers, and other observers have argued that the HIPAA Privacy Rule is not sufficient for the task and may, in fact, have the unintended consequence of undermining public health research. At the request of the U.S. Department of Health and Human Services (HHS) and a number of private groups, the IOM reviewed the rule's track record.

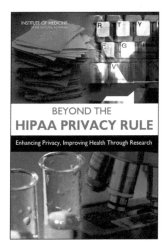

Beyond the HIPAA Privacy Rule: Enhancing Privacy, Improving Health Through Research (2009) finds that the rule does not protect privacy as well as it should, and that it impedes important health research. The report recommends that the HHS work with other federal agencies to develop an entirely new approach to protecting personal health information in research. The new framework should apply privacy, data security, and accountability standards uniformly to information used in all health-related research in the United States, regardless of who funds or conducts the research.

To aid in advancing research while protecting privacy, the new framework should facilitate the use of health data in which personally identifiable information is removed and provide legal sanctions against unauthorized reidentification of individuals. In addition, the framework should provide ethical oversight of research in which use of personally identifiable information without individual consent is necessary, enlisting local ethical review boards to assess proposed projects on a case-by-case basis. Alternatively, institutions could be certified at the federal level to carry out this kind of research, having proved they have policies and practices in place to protect data privacy.

In the event that policy makers continue to rely on the current HIPAA Privacy Rule rather than adopt the new approach, the report also provides a series of recommended changes to improve both the rule as it currently stands as well as the guidance that the HHS provides for complying with it.

Designing better HIV intervention trials

In the more than 25 years since HIV was discovered, researchers have made significant strides in identifying effective prevention interventions. Yet the epidemic continues to expand. With an estimated 2.5 million new HIV infections occurring globally each year, efforts are needed to make better use of existing HIV prevention strategies and to identify new ones. In particular, women need additional methods for preventing HIV, given the many women who become infected under circumstances not under their control.

With an estimated 2.5 million new HIV infections occurring globally each year, efforts are needed to make better use of existing HIV prevention strategies and to identify new ones.

A near-perfect biomedical intervention for preventing HIV infection is unlikely to be available in the near future. New methods currently in late-stage clinical trials are likely to offer modest levels of protection, and perhaps only in specific circumstances. For this and other reasons, researchers have found it difficult to determine whether or not methods or products being tested actually provide useful levels of protection against HIV infection, and precisely how much protection they offer. At the request of the Bill & Melinda Gates Foundation, the IOM examined how best to meet this challenge.

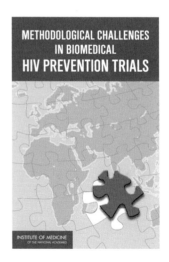

Methodological Challenges in Biomedical HIV Prevention Trials (2008) presents a coordinated set of steps for improving the design, monitoring, and analysis of late-stage clinical trials of various types of interventions, excluding vaccines. In sum, the report concludes that alternative trial designs, more extensive site preparation, and careful monitoring and analysis of trial results are critical in evaluating prevention interventions and determining which of them can exert the greatest possible long-term impact on the HIV epidemic.

**Biomedical Approaches to HIV Prevention
Tested in Late-Stage Efficacy Trials**

Male circumcision, or removal of the penile foreskin, has been shown to reduce the risk of HIV infection in men.

Microbicides are topical substances applied to the vagina or rectum that can potentially prevent HIV.

Pre-exposure prophylaxis, employing antiretroviral drugs used for HIV treatment, may help prevent HIV infection..

Cervical barriers were hypothesized to protect women from HIV by covering the cervix and blocking the upper genital tract, which is more vulnerable to HIV infection.

Suppression of HSV-2, the primary cause of genital herpes, may help reduce sexual acquisition and transmission of HIV.

Vaccines may enhance the body's immune defenses to prevent HIV infection.

SOURCE: Methodological Challenges in Biomedical HIV Prevention Trials, p. 3.

Assessing government research programs

The National Institute for Occupational Safety and Health (NIOSH) is one of the key agencies charged with protecting the well-being of millions of workers nationwide who face potential dangers on their jobs. As part of its effort to establish and evaluate performance measures for each of its research programs, NIOSH requested that the National Research Council and the IOM review the performance of a number of its research programs and suggest emerging issues that should be studied in order to achieve future improvements in worker protection. The first report was issued in 2006, on hearing loss prevention, and eight additional reports in the series *Reviews of Research Programs of the National Institute for Occupational Safety and Health* have since been released. For each program, a key challenge is determining how to obtain maximum scientific and social pay-offs.

Traumatic Injury Research at NIOSH (2008) reviews the agency's research conducted between 1996 and 2005 on this type of injury, defined as "any damage inflicted to the body by energy transfer during work with a short duration between exposure and health event." In sum, the report finds that the research program focused on the correct priority areas and yielded important gains in protecting workers' safety. In addition, the program's stated strategic goals for future research correctly target major contributors to occupational injuries and deaths and adequately consider populations and groups of workers who are at disproportionate risk.

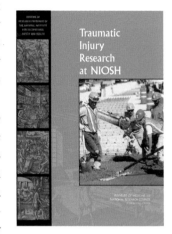

The report offers nine recommendations to help NIOSH build on its success. Among them, the agency should work with other federal agencies that support injury prevention and control research to outline fruitful areas of collaboration; develop a strategic plan for evaluating its research-to-practice efforts and for building the capacity to carry out these efforts; and expand research on the safety impacts of changes in the nature of work and on interventions intended to improve organization policies and practices.

**Goals and Subgoals of the NIOSH
Traumatic Injury Research Program**[a]

1. **Reduce injuries and fatalities due to motor vehicles**
    1.1. Reduce occupational injuries and fatalities due to highway motor vehicle crashes
    1.2. Reduce occupational injuries and fatalities due to motor vehicle incidents in highway and street construction work zones
2. **Reduce injuries and fatalities due to falls from elevations**
    2.1. Reduce worker falls from roofs
    2.2. Improve fall-arrest harnesses
    2.3. Reduce worker falls from telecommunications towers

continued

Continued

3. **Reduce injuries and fatalities due to workplace violence**
4. **Reduce injuries and fatalities due to machines**
   4.1. Reduce injuries and deaths caused by tractor rollovers by increasing availability and use of effective rollover protective structures
   4.2. Reduce worker injuries and deaths caused by paper balers
   4.3. Reduce injuries and deaths caused by machines through the conduct of fatality investigations and the dissemination of prevention strategies
5. **Reduce acute back injury**
   5.1. Reduce acute injuries caused by patient handling
   5.2. Evaluate interventions used to prevent acute injuries caused by material handling
6. **Reduce injuries and fatalities among workers in Alaska**
   6.1. Reduce injuries and fatalities in commercial fishing
   6.2. Reduce injuries and fatalities in helicopter logging operations
   6.3. Reduce injuries and fatalities in Alaska aviation
7. **Reduce injuries and fatalities to emergency responders**
   7.1. Reduce injuries and fatalities to firefighters
   7.2. Improve protection for ambulance workers in patient compartments
   7.3. Improve protection for emergency workers responding to large-scale disasters and terrorist attacks
8. **Reduce injuries and fatalities to working youth**
   8.1. Influence legislative changes to protect young workers
   8.2. Reduce child agricultural injuries
   8.3. Foster the development and widespread use of safety materials and intervention strategies to protect young workers

[a]The numbering of the goals here is consistent with the numbering of the goals as presented in the evidence package prepared by NIOSH for the committee. The numbering is not a ranking of goals by research priority.

SOURCE: Traumatic Injury Research at NIOSH, p. 4.

The Personal Protective Technology Program at NIOSH (2008) reviews the agency's research conducted between 2001 and 2007 on the safety gear that its regulations require workers to wear. Such equipment includes respirators worn by construction workers and miners to protect against exposure to silica, dust, and hazardous gases; protective clothing, respirators, and gloves worn by firefighters and mine rescue workers to avoid burns and smoke inhalation; and respirators and protective clothing worn by health care workers to prevent acquiring an infectious disease. The report finds that overall, the research program made meaningful contributions to improving worker health and safety, correctly focused on areas of highest priority, and incorporated efforts to translate research results into products and processes that have proved useful in the workplace.

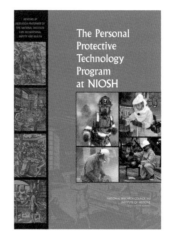

**Personal Protective Technology Program
Strategic Goals and Objectives**

Strategic Goal 1: Reduce Exposure to Inhalation Hazards

Objective 1.   Ensure the integrity of the national inventory of respirators through the implementation of a just-in-time respirator certification process.

Objective 2.   Develop CBRN respirator standards to reduce exposure to CBRN threats.

Objective 3.   Ensure the availability of mine emergency respirators for escape from mines.

Objective 4.   Improve reliability and level of protection by developing criteria that influence personal protective equipment designs to better fit the range of facial dimensions of respirator users in the U.S. workforce.

continued

Continued

Objective 5.   Quantify the impacts of various personal protective equipment on viral transmission.

Objective 6.   Evaluate the nanofiber-based fabrics and NIOSH-certified respirators for respiratory protection against nanoparticles.

Objective 7.   Develop and make available end-of-service-life indicator technologies that reliably sense or model performance to ensure respirator users receive effective respiratory protection.

Objective 8.   Gather information on the use of respirators in the workplace to identify research, intervention, and outreach needs.

Strategic Goal 2: Reduce Exposure to Dermal Hazards

Objective 1.   Improve chemical-barrier protective clothing testing and use practices to reduce worker exposure to chemical dermal hazards.

Objective 2.   Improve emergency responder protective clothing to reduce exposure to thermal, biological, and chemical dermal hazards.

Objective 3.   Investigate physiological and ergonomic impact of protective ensembles on individual wearers in affecting worker exposure to dermal hazards.

Strategic Goal 3: Reduce Exposure to Injury Hazards*

Objective 1.   Develop and evaluate warning devices for fire services.

NOTE: CBRN = chemical, biological, radiological, and nuclear.

*The PPT Program has additional objectives under this strategic goal that are related to hearing protection, protection from falls, and antivibration technologies. These objectives are not the focus of this review; some aspects of these objectives have been discussed in other National Academies' reviews.

SOURCE: The Personal Protective Technology Program at NIOSH, p. 4.

In advancing its mission, NIOSH should push to implement a 2001 congressional mandate that calls for developing a comprehensive state-of-the-art federal program focused on personal protective technology. Among other steps, the agency should establish extramural research centers of excellence; expedite the revision of respirator certification regulations; increase research on human factors, including individual behaviors and organizational behaviors, that influence workers' use of protective equipment; and emphasize pre- and postmarket testing of protective products.

Beyond providing guidance to help protect workers on the ground, IOM committees also have taken on the task of safeguarding the health of workers in space. As part of its quest to expand humanity's reach into the cosmos, the National Aeronautics and Space Administration (NASA) is preparing to send astronauts on various sorts of long-duration flights beyond low Earth orbit. These voyagers will face a complex set of safety and health hazards that result from the often-harsh space environment and the limits of available in-mission medical care. In determining its plans, NASA has asked the IOM for advice on a number of matters. Based on this advice, NASA has developed a new process to ensure that it gives proper attention to the full range of potential human health risks. From this effort, the agency has compiled a series of 25 "evidence books" that encapsulate the health-risk evidence gathered from both scientific studies and spaceflight experiences. Again, NASA turned to the IOM to evaluate the content of the evidence books and the process that the agency used in selecting which risks to explore.

Review of NASA's Human Research Program Evidence Books: A Letter Report (2008) concludes that the agency has developed a thorough and well-conceived framework for documenting the evidence base, establishing research priorities, and integrating research findings into occupational health and safety measures for the space crew. The report also offers a number of recommendations to help NASA strengthen the content, composition, and dissemination of the evidence books. One key step will be to update the books continuously to reflect the most up-to-date information available. In this way, the cumulative knowledge base will best serve the interests of mission planners, researchers, and ultimately the individuals who will face the risks in their role as space travelers.

Looking toward tomorrow

In addition to facing issues with immediate import, the nation's research enterprise and the policy makers who shape it must pay sharp attention to new and emerging challenges—and opportunities. The IOM helps to identify and illuminate these emerging challenges.

Understanding the brain

Neuroscience has made phenomenal advances over the past 50 years, and the pace of discovery continues to accelerate. Such prospects led the IOM's Forum on Neuroscience and Nervous Systems Disorders to convene a workshop in which participants from diverse fields would examine emerging insights and, as an ultimate goal, excite both the scientific community and the public about the richness of knowledge that neuroscience is providing.

From Molecules to Minds: Challenges for the 21st Century: Workshop Summary (2008) explores the latest achievements, and remaining challenges, in deciphering the inner workings of that most complicated

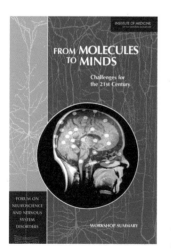

and exquisite organ—the brain. Researchers have crafted gains by combining past knowledge with information obtained using a host of new tools, including neuronal "light switches" and computer learning technologies. In light of such collective advances, numerous participants argued that neuroscience is on the cusp of even greater transformational progress in plotting how the brain operates and how its operations result in mental activity.

Looking ahead, participants discussed three "Grand Challenges" that neuroscientists, working in tandem with researchers in a number of related fields, might profitably consider. The first challenge centers on determining how the brain's internal activity gives rise to thought, emotion, and behavior. The second focuses on determining how biology and experience interact to shape a person's brain and make that person a unique individual. The third will involve identifying ways for people to keep their brains healthy, and especially how they can protect, restore, or enhance the functioning of their brains as they age. Such questions, having once simply been assigned to future study, now are becoming approachable in a scientifically rigorous manner.

Advancing the genomic revolution

Until recently, the sequencing of the human genome—the body's fundamental blueprint—also was thought to be purely science fiction. Yet in recent years, such sequencing has generated excitement about the potential of genomic innovations to improve medical care, preventive and community health services, and public health. Until fairly recently, physicians have been able to use a patient's genetic information in diagnosing only a few relatively rare genetic diseases, such as cystic fibrosis and Huntington's disease. But a transformation in the field is under way, and the IOM's Roundtable on Translating Genomic-Based Research for Health has held workshops to foster discussions about how genomics is changing.

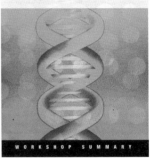
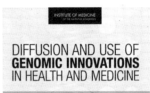

Diffusion and Use of Genomic Innovations in Health and Medicine: Workshop Summary (2008) reports on a workshop aimed at speeding the transfer of research findings to health care, public health, and health policy. The discussions centered around several key areas, including the processes or pathways by which new scientific findings in genomics move from the research setting into health care; the lessons that can be learned from the translation of other new technologies into practical application; and the practical incentives and barriers that now promote or hinder the translation of genomic advances into health care both within the United States and globally.

Innovations in Service Delivery in the Age of Genomics: Workshop Summary (2009) discussed how new discoveries in genomics are changing the way in which diseases are diagnosed and treated. Whereas previously, genetic testing could only screen for rare genetic disorders, increasingly, patients and their physicians now are able to use genetic information to predict the risk of common diseases such as diabetes and breast cancer and to help determine prevention and treatment options. Genetic specialists have long been the main providers of genetic services, offering intensive counseling for rare genetic disorders. However, as the trend shifts

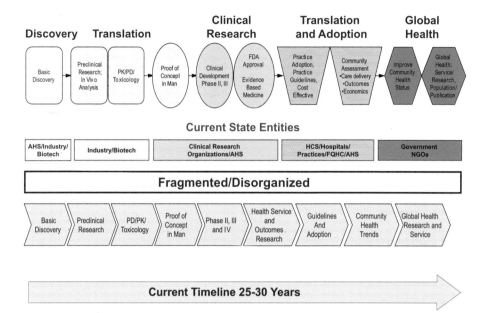

Translation of innovations.

SOURCE: Diffusion and Use of Genomic Innovations in Health and Medicine: Workshop Summary, p. 4.

from genetic testing largely being undertaken for rare genetic disorders to, increasingly, individuals being screened for common diseases, providers need to be knowledgeable about and comfortable using genetic information to improve their patients' health.

Convening and Collaborating: Forums and Roundtables

As a fundamental part of its work, the Institute of Medicine (IOM) serves as a neutral meeting place where diverse groups of people can meet to share information and advance knowledge. Although creating common ground can occur through formal committees with specific objectives and areas of study, it often takes place through forums, roundtables, and symposia that provide opportunities for serendipitous discovery and critical, cross-disciplinary thinking.

Symposia are most often held as part of the dissemination activities for an IOM report on a focused topic. A series of symposia on childhood obesity, for example, brought the subject and the IOM's report to the attention of regional media markets and stakeholders.

Forums and roundtables draw together an array of stakeholders interested in a broad area of health science or public policy for a long-term, evidence-based dialogue. Members of forums and roundtables typically include experts from the scientific and practice communities; leaders from government, academia, and industry; and representatives of consumer and public interest groups, among others.

These gatherings are intended to illuminate issues through discussion and debate across sectors and institutions rather than to make specific, actionable recommendations to directly drive policy. Bringing together these individuals can be a powerful force in creating the shared knowledge, trust, and understanding necessary to foster progress in the most difficult areas of health and science policy.

Food Forum

Since 1993, the Food Forum of the Food and Nutrition Board has engaged science and technology leaders in the food industry, top administrators

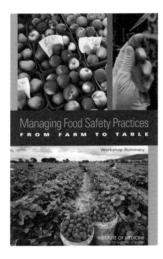

from federal agencies in the United States and Canada, top-level representatives from academia, and leaders of consumer interest groups in discussing food-related issues. The dialogue established during meetings is intended to illuminate emerging issues in the broad areas of food science, food safety, and nutrition, including technologies and regulations. The Forum's most recent workshop explored the use of nanotechnology in food and the management of food safety practices from the beginning of the supply chain to the marketplace in an effort to understand food safety risks that continue to emerge.

Forum on Drug Discovery, Development, and Translation

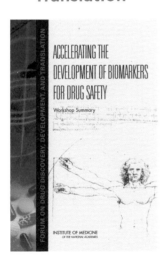

The Forum on Drug Discovery, Development, and Translation, created in 2005 by the Board on Health Sciences Policy, provides an opportunity for leaders from government, academia, industry, and other stakeholder groups to meet several times a year to discuss ongoing and emerging issues in pharmacology. In addition, the Forum commissions research papers to synthesize the literature on selected topics. Forum workshops have looked at diverse issues such as improving the process for reporting adverse drug events and advancing understanding of the benefits and risks of pharmaceuticals.

Forum on Microbial Threats

The Forum on Microbial Threats—formerly called the Forum on Emerging Infections, which was established in 1996—considers issues related to the prevention, detection, and management of infectious diseases. The Forum's membership includes individuals from a range of disciplines and organizations in the public and private sectors, including the public health, medical, pharmaceutical, veterinarian, plant pathology, academic science, agricultural, national security, and environmental communities. In recent years, Forum dialogues have illuminated priorities in infectious disease research and public health policy; the use of new scientific and policy tools; and opportunities for more effective collaboration between the private and the public sectors. Recent workshops have focused on global climate change and the emergence and spread of infectious diseases, as well as on the biological and ecological context of vector-borne diseases and their impact on the health of the public.

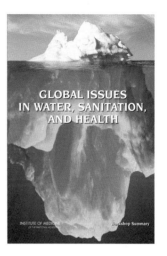

Forum on Neuroscience and Nervous System Disorders

Established in 2006, the Forum on Neuroscience and Nervous System Disorders focuses on building partnerships to further understand the brain and nervous system disorders in their structure and function and to share effective clinical prevention and treatment strategies. The Forum concentrates on six main areas: nervous system disorders, mental illness and addiction, the genetics of nervous system disorders, cognition and behavior, modeling and imaging, and ethical and social issues. The Forum brings together leaders from private-sector sponsors of biomedical and clinical research, federal agencies sponsoring and regulating biomedical and clinical research, foundations, the academic community, and public and consumer groups. The Forum's most recent workshops focused on neuroscience biomarkers and the environmental and research challenges of autism. In addition, the Forum is beginning a new initiative to focus attention on the "grand challenges" facing the neuro-

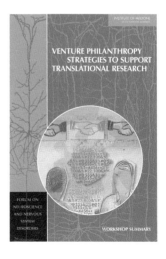

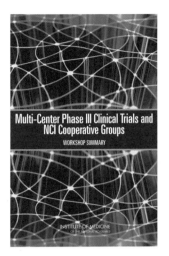

science field and the infrastructure required to meet these challenges.

National Cancer Policy Forum

The National Cancer Policy Forum was established in 2005 to succeed the National Cancer Policy Board, which had been formed in 1997. The Forum considers a range of issues in science, clinical medicine, public health, and public policy relevant to the goals of preventing, palliating, and curing cancer. The Forum's two most recent workshops examined cancer in older people and the genetic testing and counseling issues related to cancer patients.

Forum on Medical and Public Health Preparedness for Catastrophic Events

The Forum on Medical and Public Health Preparedness for Catastrophic Events, established in 2007, focuses on strengthening the nation's medical and public health preparedness for acts of terrorism or natural disasters

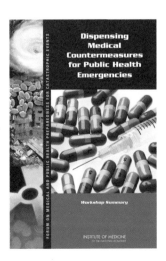

by improving communication and the coordination of activities among federal, state, and local government agencies as well as private-sector groups. The Forum, which convenes three times a year, brings together major stakeholders from government, industry, professional societies, foundations, academia, and other interested groups to discuss emerging scientific research and policy matters related to national preparedness. Among the new initiatives under development for 2009 are a workshop on medical surge capacity and a series of regional meetings devoted to exploring situational standards of care and allocation of scarce resources.

Roundtable on Health Literacy

The Roundtable on Health Literacy was created in 2004, in response to the IOM report *Health Literacy: A Prescription to End Confusion,* which found that nearly half of all American adults—90 million people—have difficulty understanding and using health information. The Roundtable brings together leaders from academia, industry, government, foundations, and patient and consumer groups who have an interest and role in improving health literacy. The Roundtable's workshops have exposed a number of specific concerns relevant to health literacy, including the organizational changes necessary to improve health literacy and the role of health literacy in transforming health care quality.

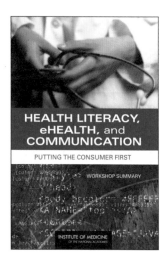

Roundtable on Environmental Health Sciences, Research, and Medicine

Established in 1998, the Roundtable on Environmental Health Sciences, Research, and Medicine brings together stakeholders from government, academia, industry, and environmental groups to discuss sensitive and difficult issues related to environmental health. The Roundtable currently has three areas of emphasis: the human-impacted environment, gene–environment interactions, and the monitoring of environmental health. Two recent Roundtable workshops have looked at the environmental public health impacts of disasters, with a focus on Hurricane Katrina, and the various aspects and economics of "green" health care institutions.

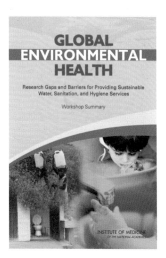

Roundtable on Evidence-Based Medicine

The Roundtable on Evidence-Based Medicine, established in 2006, focuses on examining how evidence is generated and used to improve health and

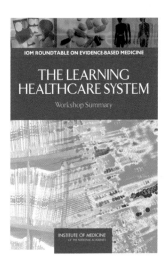

health care. In particular, the Roundtable aims to identify issues that are not being adequately considered, barriers that are impeding progress and ways to overcome those barriers, and priorities for action. Roundtable members include consumers and patients, health professionals, representatives from health care delivery organizations, evaluators and clinical researchers, employees and employers, health information technology developers, health care manufacturers, insurers, and regulators, among others. The Roundtable concentrates on three main areas: evidence development, evidence application, and sustainable capacity in the areas of clinical effectiveness research, electronic health records, best practices, and evidence communication. Several recent Roundtable workshops have focused on the *learning health care system*, and examined how the health care delivery system might better capture and apply insights generated in the course of care, as well as achieve value in health care.

Roundtable on Translating Genomic-Based Research for Health

The Roundtable on Translating Genomic-Based Research for Health focuses on advancing the field of genomics and improving the translation of research findings to health care, education, and policy. The Roundtable brings together leaders from academia, industry, government, foundations, and other groups who have a mutual interest in a range of emerging issues, including the economic implications of genomic research and its clinical applications, access to the results of genomic research, and public concerns about genomic science. To achieve its objectives, the Roundtable conducts structured discussions, workshops, and symposia. Roundtable members determine specific agenda topics, which have spanned a broad range of issues relevant to the translation process. The Roundtable has conducted workshops on the translation process that include diffusion of genomic information, innovations in genetic service delivery, and systems for research and evaluation of genetic/genomic innovations.

Roundtable on Health Disparities

The Roundtable on Health Disparities focuses on issues related to racial and ethnic disparities in health and health care as a national problem, the development of programs and strategies to reduce disparities, and the need to encourage new leadership in a variety of fields to reduce disparities. Roundtable members include experts from the health and social sciences, industry, and the community. Recent Roundtable workshops have focused on the challenges and successes in reducing health disparities.

Producing Tomorrow's Health Leaders: Fellowships at the Institute of Medicine

In addition to providing guidance on a range of health and policy issues, the Institute of Medicine (IOM) offers a number of fellowship opportunities for health professionals and behavioral and social scientists. The fellowships provide exposure to the health policy processes of Congress and the executive branch, as well as opportunities to engage with the IOM's committees and other activities.

Robert Wood Johnson Health Policy Fellowships

For more than three decades, The Robert Wood Johnson Foundation Health Policy Fellowships program has enhanced the careers of outstanding mid-career academic health professionals, community health leaders, and behavioral and social scientists. Through a unique and comprehensive orientation program designed and administered by the IOM, followed by high-level work assignments in Congress and the administration, more than 200 fellows have participated in shaping federal health policy. Strategically positioned at the nexus of health care, policy, and politics, fellows have frontline responsibilities in shaping the nation's legislation and regulations governing health and health care.

Fellows frequently have been cited by members of Congress, the administration, and the health policy community as significantly improving the outcomes of the health policy-making process. For example, Mario Pacheco (2000–2001) came to his congressional assignment with a concern about obesity in the Hispanic population and energetically supported the successful passage of legislation that created a study of school-based vending machines and their effect on childhood nutrition.

The scientific and clinical expertise that fellows possess makes valuable contributions to the deliberations of federal policy makers. Consequently, fellows are in great demand during their year in Washington, DC, and beyond. They are recruited for congressional staff positions and have taken assignments in the administration, including in the Office of the Secretary of Health and Human Services, the Department of Defense, the Office of Management and Budget, and the White House Office of Domestic Policy. Federal and state agencies, along with professional organizations and associations, also enlist alumni of this program for their insight and experience to serve in leadership roles.

Outside of government, alumni serve as university presidents, vice chancellors, and department chairs and as deans of schools of medicine, nursing, and public health. Many of them continue to enthusiastically maintain their connections to the workings of government, and some alumni have become official liaisons in government relations for their universities and professional societies. For examples, Kristofer Hagglund (2000–2001) and Karen Edison (1999–2000) are the codirectors and cofounders of the Center for Health Policy at the University of Missouri–Columbia.

IOM Anniversary Fellows Program

To celebrate its 35th anniversary in 2005, the IOM created a new fellowship program to enable talented health science scholars early in their careers to participate in the work of the IOM and to further their careers as future leaders in the health field. IOM boards, committees, and roundtables provide exceptional—and in many ways unique—learning environments that can offer early-career scholars extensive opportunities to interact with eminent researchers, policy experts, and clinicians from across the country on a range of important health issues.

The 2-year program is open to individuals who hold nontenured faculty positions in any university. It especially welcomes applications from underrepresented minority candidates. Fellows continue with their main academic responsibilities while engaging part-time in various IOM activities. A one-week immersion in the health policy arena in Washington, DC, a mentoring relationship with a senior IOM member, and a flexible research stipend enhance the value of the program. The IOM anticipates that the benefits of gaining new knowledge, professional connections, and broad exposure to policy leaders will attract an outstanding pool of applicants from a range of health-related disciplines.

An endowment from the American Board of Obstetrics and Gynecology (ABOG) has created the Norman F. Gant/American Board of Obstetrics and Gynecology Fellowship. The fellowship, created to honor Norman F. Gant, M.D., a member of the IOM and the executive director of ABOG, is targeted to obstetricians and gynecologists early in their careers.

Distinguished Nurse Scholar Program

The Distinguished Nurse Scholar Program is designed to assist outstanding nurse leaders in playing a more prominent role in health policy development at the national level. The program seeks individuals who have the capacity and skills to help increase policy makers' awareness and understanding of critical issues related to nursing. As part of the program, the scholar is asked to produce a policy-oriented paper or to become actively involved in an IOM study related to his or her area of expertise.

The program, initiated in 1992, is supported by the American Academy of Nursing and the American Nurses Foundation and is conducted by the IOM. Each year, one senior nurse scholar is selected from an eligible institution or organization to come to Washington, DC, to participate in a one-year program of orientation and work at the IOM.

Recent and Upcoming Reports

This chapter lists reports released by the Institute of Medicine from 2007 through 2009 as well as select older reports, grouped by subject area. Following the reports are upcoming reports expected to be released through 2010. A 🏛 denotes a congressionally mandated study.[1]

Recent reports (2007–2009)

Aging

Cancer in Elderly People: Workshop Proceedings, National Cancer Policy Forum, 2007.

The Development of DRIs 1994–2004: Lessons Learned and New Challenges: Workshop Summary, Food and Nutrition Board, 2007.

🏛 **Improving the Quality of Long-Term Care,** Health Care Services, 2000.

Improving the Social Security Disability Decision Process, Military and Veterans Health, 2007.

The National Children's Study Research Plan: A Review, Board on Children, Youth, and Families, IOM/NRC, 2008.

Redesigning the Clinical Effectiveness Research Paradigm: Innovation and Practice-Based Approaches, Executive Office, 2009.

[1]The Board on the Health of Select Populations was previously known as the Board on Military and Veterans Health and Medical Follow-Up Agency; the Board on Global Health was previously known as the Board on International Health; the Board on Population Health and Public Health Practice was previously known as the Board on Health Promotion and Disease Prevention.

Retooling for an Aging America: Building the Health Care Workforce, Health Care Services, 2008.

Violence Prevention in Low- and Middle-Income Countries: Finding a Place on the Global Agenda: Workshop Summary, Global Health, 2008.

Biomedical and health research

Accelerating Development of Biomarkers for Drug Safety: Workshop Summary, Health Sciences Policy, 2009.

Addressing the Barriers to Pediatric Drug Development: Workshop Summary, Health Sciences Policy, 2008.

Addressing the Threat of Drug Resistant Tuberculosis: A Realistic Assessment of the Challenges: Workshop Summary, Health Sciences Policy, 2009.

Assessing the Medical Risks of Oocyte Donation for Stem Cell Research: Workshop Report, Health Sciences Policy, 2007.

Assessment of Future Scientific Needs for Live Variola Virus, Global Health, 2009.

Assessment of the NIOSH Head-and-Face Anthropometric Survey of U.S. Respirator Users, Health Sciences Policy, 2008.

Autism and the Environment: Challenges and Opportunities for Research: Workshop Proceedings, Health Sciences Policy, 2007.

Beyond the HIPAA Privacy Rule: Enhancing Privacy, Improving Health Through Research, Health Sciences Policy, 2009.

Breakthrough Business Models: Drug Development for Rare and Neglected Diseases and Individualized Therapies: Workshop Summary, Health Sciences Policy, 2009.

Conflict of Interest in Medical Research, Education, and Practice, Health Sciences Policy, 2009.

The Development of DRIs 1994–2004: Lessons Learned and New Challenges: Workshop Summary, Food and Nutrition Board, 2007.

Diffusion and Use of Genomic Innovations in Health and Medicine: Workshop Summary, Health Sciences Policy, 2008.

Dispensing Medical Countermeasures for Public Health Emergencies: Workshop Summary, Health Sciences Policy, 2008.

Effectiveness of National Biosurveillance Systems: BioWatch and the Public Health System, Interim Report, Health Sciences Policy, 2009.

Emerging Safety Science: Workshop Summary, Health Sciences Policy, 2008.

Ethical Considerations for Research Involving Prisoners, Health Sciences Policy, 2007.

Evidence-Based Medicine and the Changing Nature of Healthcare: Workshop Summary, Executive Office, 2008.

Examining the Health Disparities Research Plan of the National Institutes of Health: Unfinished Business, Health Sciences Policy, 2006.

Foodborne Disease and Public Health: An Iranian-American Workshop, Food and Nutrition Board, 2008.

From Molecules to Minds: Challenges for the 21st Century: Workshop Summary, Health Sciences Policy, 2008.

The Future of Disability in America, Health Sciences Policy, 2007.

The Future of Drug Safety: Promoting and Protecting the Health of the Public, Population Health and Public Health Practice, 2007.

Genes, Behavior, and the Social Environment: Moving Beyond the Nature/Nurture Debate, Health Sciences Policy, 2006.

Global Environmental Health: Research Gaps and Barriers for Providing Sustainable Water, Sanitation, and Hygiene Services, Population Health and Public Health Practice, 2009.

Globalization, Biosecurity, and the Future of the Life Sciences, Global Health, 2006.

Guidelines for Human Embryonic Stem Cell Research, Health Sciences Policy, 2005.

Immunization Safety Review: SV40 Contamination of Polio Vaccine and Cancer, Health Promotion and Disease Prevention, 2002.

Immunization Safety Review: Thimerosal-Containing Vaccines and Neurodevelopmental Disorders, Health Promotion and Disease Prevention, 2001.

Improving the Quality of Cancer Clinical Trials: Workshop Summary, National Cancer Policy Forum, 2008.

Improving the Quality of Health Care for Mental and Substance-Use Conditions: Quality Chasm Series, Health Care Services, 2006.

Knowing What Works in Health Care: A Roadmap for the Nation, Health Care Services, 2008.

Making Better Drugs for Children with Cancer, National Cancer Policy Board, 2005.

Marijuana and Medicine: Assessing the Science Base, Neuroscience and Behavioral Health, 1999.

Marijuana as Medicine?: The Science Beyond the Controversy, Neuroscience and Behavioral Health, 2000.

Microbial Threats to Health: The Threat of Pandemic Influenza, Global Health, 2006.

Nanotechnology in Food Products: Impact on Food Science, Nutrition, and the Consumer: Workshop Summary, Food and Nutrition Board, 2009.

Neuroscience Biomarkers and Biosignatures: Converging Technologies, Emerging Partnerships: Workshop Summary, Health Sciences Policy, 2008.

Organ Donation: Opportunities for Action, Health Sciences Policy, 2006.

The Personal Protective Technology Program at NIOSH, Health Sciences Policy, 2008.

Posttraumatic Stress Disorder: Diagnosis and Assessment, Population Health and Public Health Practice, 2006.

Preterm Birth: Causes, Consequences, and Prevention, Health Sciences Policy, 2007.

Redesigning the Clinical Effectiveness Research Paradigm: Innovation and Practice-Based Approaches, Executive Office, 2009.

Research Priorities in Emergency Preparedness and Response for Public Health Systems: A Letter Report, Health Sciences Policy, 2008.

Reusability of Facemasks During an Influenza Pandemic: Facing the Flu, Health Sciences Policy, 2006.

Review of NASA's Human Research Program Evidence Books: Letter Report, Health Sciences Policy, 2008.

Safe Medical Devices for Children, Health Sciences Policy, 2005.

Science, Evolution, and Creationism, Executive Office, 2008.

Sleep Disorders and Sleep Deprivation: An Unmet Public Health Problem, Health Sciences Policy, 2006.

Spinal Cord Injury: Progress, Promise, and Priorities, Health Sciences Policy, 2005.

Use of Dietary Supplements by Military Personnel, Food and Nutrition Board, 2008.

Venture Philanthropy Strategies to Support Translational Research: Workshop Summary, Health Sciences Policy, 2009.

Children and families

Addressing the Barriers to Pediatric Drug Development: Workshop Summary, Health Sciences Policy, 2008.

Adolescent Health Services: Missing Opportunities, Board on Children, Youth, and Families, IOM/NRC, 2008.

America's Health Care Safety Net: Revisiting the 2000 IOM Report, Health Care Services, 2007.

Autism and the Environment: Challenges and Opportunities for Research: Workshop Proceedings, Health Sciences Policy, 2007.

Cancer Care for the Whole Patient: Meeting Psychosocial Health Needs, Health Care Services, 2007.

Challenges in Adolescent Health Care: Workshop Report, Board on Children, Youth, and Families, IOM/NRC, 2007.

Childhood Obesity Prevention: Actions for Local Governments, Food and Nutrition Board, 2009.

Community Perspectives on Obesity Prevention in Children: Workshop Summary, Food and Nutrition Board, 2008.

Confronting Chronic Neglect: The Education and Training of Health Professionals on Family Violence, Board on Children, Youth, and Families, IOM/NRC, 2001.

The Development of DRIs 1994–2004: Lessons Learned and New Challenges: Workshop Summary, Food and Nutrition Board, 2007.

Early Childhood Assessment: Why, What, and How, Board on Children, Youth, and Families, IOM/NRC, 2008.

Emergency Care for Children: Growing Pains, Health Care Services, 2007.

Food Marketing to Children and Youth: Threat or Opportunity? Food and Nutrition Board, 2005.

Foodborne Disease and Public Health: An Iranian-American Workshop, Food and Nutrition Board, 2008.

From Neurons to Neighborhoods: The Science of Early Childhood Development, Board on Children, Youth, and Families, IOM/NRC, 2000.

Health Insurance Is a Family Matter, Health Care Services, 2002.

Immunization Safety Review: Hepatitis B Vaccine and Demyelinating Neurological Disorders, Health Promotion and Disease Prevention, 2002.

Immunization Safety Review: Measles-Mumps-Rubella Vaccine and Autism, Health Promotion and Disease Prevention, 2001.

Immunization Safety Review: Multiple Immunizations and Immune Dysfunction, Health Promotion and Disease Prevention, 2002.

Immunization Safety Review: SV40 Contamination of Polio Vaccine and Cancer, Health Promotion and Disease Prevention, 2002.

Immunization Safety Review: Thimerosal-Containing Vaccines and Neurodevelopmental Disorders, Health Promotion and Disease Prevention, 2001.

Investing in Children's Health: A Community Approach to Addressing Health Disparities: Workshop Summary, Population Health and Public Health Practice, 2009.

The National Children's Study Research Plan: A Review, Board on Children, Youth, and Families, IOM/NRC, 2008.

Nutrition Standards and Meal Requirements for National School Lunch and Breakfast Programs: Phase I. Proposed Approach for Recommending Revisions, Food and Nutrition Board, 2008.

Nutrition Standards for Foods in Schools: Leading the Way Toward Healthier Youth, Food and Nutrition Board, 2007.

Preterm Birth: Causes, Consequences, and Prevention, Health Sciences Policy, 2007.

Preventing Childhood Obesity: Health in the Balance, Food and Nutrition Board and Board on Health Promotion and Disease Prevention, 2005.

Preventing Mental, Emotional, and Behavioral Disorders Among Young People: Progress and Possibilities, Board on Children, Youth, and Families, IOM/NRC, 2009.

Preventing Teen Motor Crashes: Contributions from the Behavioral and Social Sciences, Board on Children, Youth, and Families, IOM/NRC/Transportation Research Board, 2007.

Progress in Preventing Childhood Obesity: How Do We Measure Up? Food and Nutrition Board, 2007.

Redesigning the Clinical Effectiveness Research Paradigm: Innovation and Practice-Based Approaches, Executive Office, 2009.

Violence Prevention in Low- and Middle-Income Countries: Finding a Place on the Global Agenda: Workshop Summary, Global Health, 2008.

WIC Food Packages: Time for a Change, Food and Nutrition Board, 2005.

Diseases

Achieving Sustainable Global Capacity for Surveillance and Response to Emerging Diseases of Zoonotic Origin: Workshop Report, Global Health, 2008.

Addressing the Threat of Drug Resistant Tuberculosis: A Realistic Assessment of the Challenges: Workshop Summary, Health Sciences Policy, 2009.

Antivirals for Pandemic Influenza: Guidance on Developing a Distribution and Dispensing Program, Population Health and Public Health Practice, 2008.

Assessing and Improving Value of Cancer Treatment: Workshop Summary, Health Care Services, 2009.

Assessing the Quality of Cancer Care: An Approach to Measurement in Georgia, National Cancer Policy Board, 2005.

Assessment of the Role of Intermittent Preventive Treatment for Malaria in Infants: Letter Report, Global Health, 2008.

BioWatch and Public Health Surveillance: Evaluating Systems for the Early Detection of Biological Threats, Health Sciences Policy, 2009.

Cancer Care for the Whole Patient: Meeting Psychosocial Health Needs, Health Care Services, 2007.

Design Considerations for Evaluating the Impact of PEPFAR: Workshop Summary, Global Health, 2008.

The Development of DRIs 1994–2004: Lessons Learned and New Challenges: Workshop Summary, Food and Nutrition Board, 2007.

Ensuring Quality Cancer Care Through the Oncology Workforce: Sustaining Care in the 21st Century: Workshop Summary, National Cancer Policy Forum, 2009.

Food Marketing to Children and Youth: Threat or Opportunity? Food and Nutrition Board, 2005.

Foodborne Disease and Public Health: An Iranian-American Workshop, Food and Nutrition Board, 2008.

From Cancer Patient to Cancer Survivor: Lost in Transition, National Cancer Policy Board, 2005.

Global Climate Change and Extreme Weather Events: Understanding the Potential Contributions to the Emergence, Reemergence, and Spread of Infectious Disease: Workshop Summary, Global Health, 2008.

Global Infectious Disease Surveillance and Detection: Assessing the Challenges: Workshop Summary, Global Health, 2007.

Implementing Cancer Survivorship Care Planning: Workshop Summary, National Cancer Policy Forum, 2006.

Implementing Colorectal Cancer Screening: Workshop Summary, National Cancer Policy Forum, 2008.

Improving the Quality of Cancer Clinical Trials: Workshop Summary, National Cancer Policy Forum, 2008.

Learning from SARS: Preparing for the Next Disease Outbreak: Workshop Summary, Global Health, 2004.

Marijuana and Medicine: Assessing the Science Base, Neuroscience and Behavioral Health, 1999.

Methodological Challenges in Biomedical HIV Prevention Trials, Global Health, 2008.

Microbial Evolution and Co-Adaptation: A Tribute to the Life and Scientific Legacies of Joshua Lederberg: Workshop Summary, Global Health, 2009.

Multi-Center Phase III Clinical Trials and NCI Cooperative Groups: Workshop Summary, National Cancer Policy Forum, 2009.

The National Children's Study Research Plan: A Review, Board on Children, Youth, and Families, 2008.

Preventing Childhood Obesity: Health in the Balance, Food and Nutrition, Board and Board on Health Promotion and Disease Prevention, 2005.

Redesigning the Clinical Effectiveness Research Paradigm: Innovation and Practice-Based Approaches, Executive Office, 2009.

Reusability of Facemasks During an Influenza Pandemic: Facing the Flu, Health Sciences Policy, 2006.

Sustaining Global Surveillance and Response to Emerging Zoonotic Diseases, Global Health, 2009.

Use of Dietary Supplements by Military Personnel, Food and Nutrition Board, 2008.

The Utility of Proximity-Based Herbicide Exposure Assessment in Epidemiologic Studies of Vietnam Veterans, Military and Veterans Health, 2008.

Vector-Borne Diseases: Understanding the Environmental, Human Health, and Ecological Connections: Workshop Summary, Global Health, 2008.

Environmental health

Assessment of the NIOSH Head-and-Face Anthropometric Survey of U.S. Respirator Users, Health Sciences Policy, 2007.

Assessment of the NIOSH Head-and-Face Anthropometric Survey of U.S. Respirator Users, Health Sciences Policy, 2008.

Autism and the Environment: Challenges and Opportunities for Research: Workshop Proceedings, Health Sciences Policy, 2007.

BioWatch and Public Health Surveillance: Evaluating Systems for the Early Detection of Biological Threats, Health Sciences Policy, 2009.

The Development of DRIs 1994–2004: Lessons Learned and New Challenges: Workshop Summary, Food and Nutrition Board, 2007.

Effectiveness of National Biosurveillance Systems: BioWatch and the Public Health System, Interim Report, Health Sciences Policy, 2009.

Environmental Health Sciences Decision Making: Risk Management, Evidence, and Ethics: Workshop Summary, Population Health and Public Health Practice, 2009.

Environmental Public Health Impacts of Disasters: Hurricane Katrina: Workshop Summary, Population Health and Public Health Practice, 2007.

Foodborne Disease and Public Health: An Iranian-American Workshop, Food and Nutrition Board, 2008.

Genes, Behavior, and the Social Environment: Moving Beyond the Nature/Nurture Debate, Health Sciences Policy, 2006.

Global Environmental Health: Research Gaps and Barriers for Providing Sustainable Water, Sanitation, and Hygiene Services, Population Health and Public Health Practice, 2009.

Global Environmental Health in the 21st Century: From Governmental Regulation to Corporate Social Responsibility: Workshop Summary, Population Health and Public Health Practice, 2007.

Green Healthcare Institutions; Health, Environment, and Economics: Workshop Summary, Population Health and Public Health Practice, 2007.

Gulf War and Health, Volume 1: Depleted Uranium, Sarin, Pyridostigmine Bromide, and Vaccines, Health Promotion and Disease Prevention, 2000.

Gulf War and Health, Volume 3: Fuels, Combustion Products, and Propellants, Board on Health Promotion and Disease Prevention, 2005.

The National Children's Study Research Plan: A Review, Board on Children, Youth, and Families, 2008.

Implications of Nanotechnology for Environmental Health Research: Workshop Summary, Population Health and Public Health Practice, 2005.

Review of ATSDR's Great Lakes Report Drafts: Letter Report, Population Health and Public Health Practice, 2008.

Use of Dietary Supplements by Military Personnel, Food and Nutrition Board, 2008.

Food and nutrition

Addressing Foodborne Threats to Health: Policies, Practices, and Global Coordination, Workshop Summary, Global Health, 2006.

Childhood Obesity Prevention: Actions for Local Governments, Food and Nutrition Board, 2009.

Community Perspectives on Obesity Prevention in Children: Workshop Summary, Food and Nutrition Board, 2008.

The Development of DRIs 1994–2004: Lessons Learned and New Challenges: Workshop Summary, Food and Nutrition Board, 2007.

Dietary Reference Intakes: Proposed Definition of Dietary Fiber, Food and Nutrition Board, 2001.

Dietary Reference Intakes: The Essential Guide to Nutrient Requirements, Food and Nutrition Board, 2006.

Dietary Reference Intakes for Calcium, Phosphorus, Magnesium, Vitamin D, and Fluoride, Food and Nutrition Board, 1997.

Dietary Reference Intakes for Energy, Carbohydrate, Fiber, Fat, Fatty Acids, Cholesterol, Protein, and Amino Acids, Food and Nutrition Board, 2002.

Dietary Reference Intakes for Thiamin, Riboflavin, Niacin, Vitamin B_6, Folate, Vitamin B_{12}, Pantothenic Acid, Biotin, and Choline, Food and Nutrition Board, 1998.

Dietary Reference Intakes for Vitamin A, Vitamin K, Arsenic, Boron, Chromium, Copper, Iodine, Iron, Manganese, Molybdenum, Nickel, Silicon, Vanadium, and Zinc, Food and Nutrition Board, 2001.

Dietary Reference Intakes for Vitamin C, Vitamin E, Selenium, and Carotenoids, Food and Nutrition Board, 2000.

Dietary Reference Intakes Research Synthesis: Workshop Summary, Food and Nutrition Board, 2007.

Dietary Risk Assessment in the WIC Program, Food and Nutrition Board, 2002.

Eat for Life: The Food and Nutrition Board's Guide to Reducing Your Risk of Chronic Disease, Food and Nutrition Board, 1992.

Ensuring Safe Food: From Production to Consumption, Food and Nutrition Board, joint with the NRC Board on Agriculture, 1998.

Food Chemicals Codex: First Supplement to the Fifth Edition, Food and Nutrition Board, 2006.

Food Marketing to Children and Youth: Threat or Opportunity? Food and Nutrition Board, 2005.

Foodborne Disease and Public Health: An Iranian-American Workshop, Food and Nutrition Board, 2008.

Integrating Employee Health: A Model Program for NASA, Food and Nutrition Board, 2005.

Joint U.S.-Mexico Workshop on Preventing Obesity in Children and Youth of Mexican Origin, Food and Nutrition Board, 2007.

Managing Food Safety Practices from Farm to Table: Workshop Summary, Food and Nutrition Board, 2009.

Nanotechnology in Food Products: Impact on Food Science, Nutrition, and the Consumer: Workshop Summary, Food and Nutrition Board, 2009.

Nutrition Standards and Meal Requirements for National School Lunch and Breakfast Programs: Phase I. Proposed Approach for Recommending Revisions, Food and Nutrition Board, 2008.

Nutrition Standards for Foods in Schools: Leading the Way Toward Healthier Youth, Food and Nutrition Board, 2007.

Preventing Childhood Obesity: Health in the Balance, Food and Nutrition Board and Board on Health Promotion and Disease Prevention, 2005.

Progress in Preventing Childhood Obesity: How Do We Measure Up? Food and Nutrition Board, 2007.

The Public Health Effects of Food Deserts: Workshop Summary, Food and Nutrition Board, 2009.

Review of the Use of Process Control Indicators in the FSIS Public Health Risk-Based Inspection System: Letter Report, Food and Nutrition Board, 2009.

Seafood Choices: Balancing Benefits and Risks, Food and Nutrition Board, 2007.

Use of Dietary Supplements by Military Personnel, Food and Nutrition Board, 2008.

Weight Gain During Pregnancy: Reexamining the Guidelines, Food and Nutrition Board, 2009.

WIC Food Packages: Time for a Change, Food and Nutrition Board, 2005.

Global health

Achieving Sustainable Global Capacity for Surveillance and Response to Emerging Diseases of Zoonotic Origin: Workshop Report, Global Health, 2008.

Addressing the Threat of Drug Resistant Tuberculosis: A Realistic Assessment of the Challenges: Workshop Summary, Health Sciences Policy, 2009.

America's Vital Interest in Global Health: Protecting Our People, Enhancing Our Economy, and Advancing Our International Interests, International Health, 1997.

Assessment of Future Scientific Needs for Live Variola Virus, Global Health, 1999.

Assessment of Future Scientific Needs for Live Variola Virus, Global Health, 2009.

Assessment of the Role of Intermittent Preventive Treatment for Malaria in Infants, Letter Report, Global Health, 2008.

BioWatch and Public Health Surveillance: Evaluating Systems for the Early Detection of Biological Threats, Health Sciences Policy, 2009.

Cancer Control Opportunities in Low- and Middle-Income Countries, Global Health, 2007.

Design Considerations for Evaluating the Impact of PEPFAR, Workshop Summary, Global Health, 2008.

The Development of DRIs 1994–2004: Lessons Learned and New Challenges: Workshop Summary, Food and Nutrition Board, 2007.

Emerging Infections: Microbial Threats to Health in the United States, Health Sciences Policy, 1992.

Ethical and Legal Considerations in Mitigating Pandemic Disease: Workshop Summary, Global Health, 2007.

Foodborne Disease and Public Health: An Iranian-American Workshop, Food and Nutrition Board, 2008.

Global Climate Change and Extreme Weather Events: Understanding the Potential Contributions to the Emergence, Reemergence, and Spread of Infectious Disease, Workshop Summary, Global Health, 2008.

Global Environmental Health: Research Gaps and Barriers for Providing Sustainable Water, Sanitation, and Hygiene Services, Population Health and Public Health Practice, 2009.

Global Infectious Disease Surveillance and Detection: Assessing the Challenges: Workshop Summary, Global Health, 2007.

Global Issues in Water, Sanitation, and Health: Workshop Summary, Global Health, 2009.

Globalization, Biosecurity, and the Future of the Life Sciences, Global Health, 2006.

The Impact of Globalization on Infectious Disease Emergence and Control: Exploring the Consequences and Opportunities: Workshop Summary, Global Health, 2006.

Methodological Challenges in Biomedical HIV Prevention Trials, Global Health, 2008.

Microbial Evolution and Co-Adaptation: A Tribute to the Life and Scientific Legacies of Joshua Lederberg: Workshop Summary, Global Health, 2009.

Microbial Threats to Health: The Threat of Pandemic Influenza, Global Health, 2006.

PEPFAR Implementation: Progress and Promise, Global Health, 2007.

Plan for a Short-Term Evaluation of PEPFAR Implementation: Letter Report #1, Global Health, 2006.

Quarantine Stations at Ports of Entry Protecting the Public's Health, Global Health, 2005.

Redesigning the Clinical Effectiveness Research Paradigm: Innovation and Practice-Based Approaches, Executive Office, 2009.

Sustaining Global Surveillance and Response to Emerging Zoonotic Diseases, Global Health, 2009.

The U.S. Commitment to Global Health: Recommendations for the New Administration, Global Health, 2008.

The U.S. Commitment to Global Health: Recommendations for the Public and Private Sectors, Global Health, 2009.

Use of Dietary Supplements by Military Personnel, Food and Nutrition Board, 2008.

Vector-Borne Diseases: Understanding the Environmental, Human Health, and Ecological Connections: Workshop Summary, Global Health, 2008.

Violence Prevention in Low- and Middle-Income Countries: Finding a Place on the Global Agenda: Workshop Summary, Global Health, 2008.

Health care workforce

Adverse Drug Event Reporting: The Roles of Consumers and Health Care Professionals: Workshop Summary, Health Sciences Policy, 2007.

Assessment of the NIOSH Head-and-Face Anthropometric Survey of U.S. Respirator Users, Health Sciences Policy, 2008.

Cancer Care for the Whole Patient: Meeting Psychosocial Health Needs, Health Care Services, 2007.

Challenges in Adolescent Health Care: Workshop Report, Board on Children, Youth, and Families, IOM/NRC, 2007.

Conflict of Interest in Medical Research, Education, and Practice, Health Sciences Policy, 2009.

Design Considerations for Evaluating the Impact of PEPFAR: Workshop Summary, Global Health, 2008.

The Development of DRIs 1994–2004: Lessons Learned and New Challenges: Workshop Summary, Food and Nutrition Board, 2007.

Emergency Care for Children: Growing Pains, Health Care Services, 2007.

Emergency Medical Services at the Crossroads, Health Care Services, 2007.

Ensuring Quality Cancer Care through the Oncology Workforce: Sustaining Care in the 21st Century: Workshop Summary, National Cancer Policy Forum, 2009.

The Future of the Public's Health in the 21st Century, Health Promotion and Disease Prevention, 2002.

Hospital-Based Emergency Care: At the Breaking Point, Health Care Services, 2007.

Improving the Quality of Cancer Clinical Trials: Workshop Summary, National Cancer Policy Forum, 2008.

Integrity in Scientific Research: Creating an Environment That Promotes Responsible Conduct, Institute of Medicine, IOM/NRC, 2002.

Research Priorities in Emergency Preparedness and Response for Public Health Systems: A Letter Report, Health Sciences Policy, 2008.

Resident Duty Hours: Enhancing Sleep, Supervision, and Safety, Health Care Services, 2009.

Retooling for an Aging America: Building the Health Care Workforce, Health Care Services, 2008.

The Richard and Hinda Rosenthal Lectures 2005: Next Steps Toward Higher Quality Health Care, Institute of Medicine, 2006.

The Richard and Hinda Rosenthal Lectures 2007: Transforming Today's Health Care Workforce to Meet Tomorrow's Demands, Executive Office, 2008.

Training Physicians for Public Health Careers, Population Health and Public Health Practice, 2007.

The U.S. Oral Health Workforce in the Coming Decade: Workshop Summary, Health Care Services, 2009.

Health services, coverage, and access

Advancing Quality Improvement Research: Challenges and Opportunities: Workshop Summary, Health Care Services, 2007.

America's Health Care Safety Net: Intact but Endangered, Health Policy Programs and Fellowships, 2000.

America's Health Care Safety Net: Revisiting the 2000 IOM Report, Health Care Services, 2007.

America's Uninsured Crisis: Consequences for Health and Health Care, Health Care Services, 2009.

Assessing the Quality of Cancer Care: An Approach to Measurement in Georgia, National Cancer Policy Board, 2005.

Building a Better Delivery System: A New Engineering/Health Care Partnership, Health Care Services, 2005.

Cancer Care for the Whole Patient: Meeting Psychosocial Health Needs, Health Care Services, 2007.

Challenges in Adolescent Health Care: Workshop Report, Board on Children, Youth, and Families, IOM/NRC, 2007.

Crossing the Quality Chasm: A New Health System for the 21st Century, Committee on Quality of Health Care in America, 2001.

The Development of DRIs 1994–2004: Lessons Learned and New Challenges: Workshop Summary, Food and Nutrition Board, 2007.

Emergency Care for Children: Growing Pains, Health Care Services, 2007.

Emergency Medical Services: At the Crossroads, Health Care Services, 2007.

📖 **Epidemiologic Studies of Veterans Exposed to Depleted Uranium: Feasibility and Design Issues,** Population Health and Public Health Practice, 2008.

Evidence-Based Medicine and the Changing Nature of Healthcare: Workshop Summary, Executive Office, 2008.

📖 **Gulf War and Health: Updated Literature Review of Depleted Uranium,** Population Health and Public Health Practice, 2008.

📖 **Gulf War and Health, Volume 7: Long-term Consequences of Traumatic Brain Injury,** Population Health and Public Health Practice, 2008.

HHS in the 21st Century: Charting a New Course for a Healthier America, Executive Office, 2008.

📖 **Hospital-Based Emergency Care: At the Breaking Point,** Health Care Services, 2007.

Implementing Colorectal Cancer Screening: Workshop Summary, National Cancer Policy Forum, 2008.

Improving the Quality of Health Care for Mental and Substance-Use Conditions: Quality Chasm Series, Health Care Services, 2006.

Knowing What Works in Health Care: A Roadmap for the Nation, Health Care Services, 2008.

The Learning Healthcare System: Workshop Summary, Institute of Medicine, 2007.

📖 **Medicare's Quality Improvement Organization Program: Maximizing Potential,** Health Care Services, 2006.

The National Children's Study Research Plan: A Review, Board on Children, Youth, and Families, 2008.

Opportunities for Coordination and Clarity to Advance the National Health Information Agenda: A Brief Assessment of the Office of the National Coordinator for Health Information Technology: Letter Report, Health Care Services, 2007.

📖 **Performance Measurement: Accelerating Improvement,** Health Care Services, 2006.

📖 **Preventing Medication Errors: Quality Chasm Series,** Health Care Services, 2006.

Resident Duty Hours: Enhancing Sleep, Supervision, and Safety, Health Care Services, 2009.

Retooling for an Aging America: Building the Health Care Workforce, Health Care Services, 2008.

Rewarding Provider Performance: Aligning Incentives in Medicare, Health Care Services, 2007.

The Right Thing to Do, The Smart Thing to Do: Enhancing Diversity in Health Professions—Summary of the Symposium on Diversity in Health Professions in Honor of Herbert W. Nickens, M.D., Institute of Medicine, 2001.

Summit on Integrative Medicine and the Health of the Public: Workshop Summary, Executive Office, 2009.

To Err Is Human: Building a Safer Health System, Health Care Services, 2000.

Training Physicians for Public Health Careers, Population Health and Public Health Practice, 2007.

Unequal Treatment: Confronting Racial and Ethnic Disparities in Health Care, Health Sciences Policy, 2002.

Use of Dietary Supplements by Military Personnel, Food and Nutrition Board, 2008.

Valuing Health for Regulatory Cost-Effectiveness Analysis, Health Care Services, 2006.

Public health

Addressing the Barriers to Pediatric Drug Development: Workshop Summary, Health Sciences Policy, 2008.

Adolescent Health Services: Missing Opportunities, Board on Children, Youth, and Families, IOM/NRC, 2008.

Antivirals for Pandemic Influenza: Guidance on Developing a Distribution and Dispensing Program, Population Health and Public Health Practice, 2008.

Asbestos: Selected Cancers, Population Health and Public Health Practice, 2006.

Assessing Medical Preparedness to Respond to a Terrorist Nuclear Event: Workshop Report, Health Sciences Policy, 2009.

Assessment of Future Scientific Needs for Live Variola Virus, Global Health, 1999.

Assessment of the Role of Intermittent Preventive Treatment for Malaria in Infants: Letter Report, Global Health, 2008.

Autism and the Environment: Challenges and Opportunities for Research: Workshop Proceedings, Health Sciences Policy, 2007.

Challenges and Successes in Reducing Health Disparities: Workshop Summary, Population Health and Public Health Practice, 2008.

Challenges in Adolescent Health Care: Workshop Report, Board on Children, Youth, and Families, 2007.

The Development of DRIs 1994–2004: Lessons Learned and New Challenges: Workshop Summary, Food and Nutrition Board, 2007.

Diffusion and Use of Genomic Innovations in Health and Medicine: Workshop Summary, Health Sciences Policy, 2008.

Dispensing Medical Countermeasures for Public Health Emergencies: Workshop Summary, Health Sciences Policy, 2008.

Effectiveness of National Biosurveillance Systems: BioWatch and the Public Health System: Interim Report, Health Sciences Policy, 2009.

Emerging Safety Science, Workshop Summary, Health Sciences Policy, 2008.

Ending the Tobacco Problem: A Blueprint for the Nation, Population Health and Public Health Practice, 2007.

Ensuring Safe Food From Production to Consumption, Food and Nutrition Board, 1998.

Environmental Health Sciences Decision Making: Risk Management, Evidence, and Ethics: Workshop Summary, Population Health and Public Health Practice, 2009.

Ethical and Legal Considerations in Mitigating Pandemic Disease: Workshop Summary, Global Health, 2007.

Evaluating Occupational Health and Safety Research Programs: Evaluation Framework and Next Steps, Health Sciences Policy, 2009.

Foodborne Disease and Public Health: An Iranian-American Workshop, Food and Nutrition Board, 2008.

The Future of Drug Safety: Promoting and Protecting the Health of the Public, Population Health and Public Health Practice, 2007.

The Future of the Public's Health in the 21st Century, Health Promotion and Disease Prevention, 2002.

Global Climate Change and Extreme Weather Events: Understanding the Potential Contributions to the Emergence, Reemergence, and Spread of Infectious Disease: Workshop Summary, Global Health, 2008.

Global Environmental Health: Research Gaps and Barriers for Providing Sustainable Water, Sanitation, and Hygiene Services, Population Health and Public Health Practice, 2009.

Global Infectious Disease Surveillance and Detection: Assessing the Challenges: Workshop Summary, Global Health, 2007.

Immunization Safety Review: Hepatitis B Vaccine and Demyelinating Neurological Disorders, Health Promotion and Disease Prevention, 2002.

Immunization Safety Review: Measles-Mumps-Rubella Vaccine and Autism, Health Promotion and Disease Prevention, 2001.

Immunization Safety Review: Multiple Immunizations and Immune System Dysfunction, Health Promotion and Disease Prevention, 2002.

Immunization Safety Review: SV40 Contamination of Polio Vaccine and Cancer, Health Promotion and Disease Prevention, 2002.

Immunization Safety Review: Thimerosal-Containing Vaccines and Neurodevelopmental Disorders, Health Promotion and Disease Prevention, 2001.

Initial Guidance for an Update of the National Vaccine Plan: A Letter Report to the National Vaccine Program Office, Population Health and Public Health Practice, 2008.

Investing in Children's Health: A Community Approach to Addressing Health Disparities: Workshop Summary, Population Health and Public Health Practice, 2009.

Knowing What Works in Health Care: A Roadmap for the Nation, Health Care Services, 2008.

Managing Food Safety Practices from Farm to Table: Workshop Summary, Food and Nutrition Board, 2009.

Microbial Evolution and Co-Adaptation: A Tribute to the Life and Scientific Legacies of Joshua Lederberg: Workshop Summary, Global Health, 2009.

Modeling Community Containment for Pandemic Influenza: A Letter Report, Population Health and Public Health Practice, 2006.

The National Children's Study Research Plan: A Review, Board on Children, Youth, and Families, 2008.

Neuroscience Biomarkers and Biosignatures: Converging Technologies, Emerging Partnerships: Workshop Summary, Health Sciences Policy, 2008.

Opportunities for Coordination and Clarity to Advance the National Health Information Agenda: A Brief Assessment of the Office of the National Coordinator for Health Information Technology, Letter Report, Health Care Services, 2007.

The Personal Protective Technology Program at NIOSH, Health Sciences Policy, 2008.

Preterm Birth: Causes, Consequences, and Prevention, Health Sciences Policy, 2007.

Preventing Childhood Obesity: Health in the Balance, Food and Nutrition Board and Board on Health Promotion and Disease Prevention, 2005.

The Public Health Effects of Food Deserts: Workshop Summary, Food and Nutrition Board, 2009.

Public Health Risks of Disasters: Communication, Infrastructure, and Preparedness, Population Health and Public Health Practice, 2005.

Redesigning the Clinical Effectiveness Research Paradigm: Innovation and Practice-Based Approaches, Executive Office, 2009.

Research Priorities in Emergency Preparedness and Response for Public Health Systems: A Letter Report, Health Sciences Policy, 2008.

Retooling for an Aging America: Building the Health Care Workforce, Health Care Services, 2008.

Review of ATSDR's Great Lakes Report Drafts: Letter Report, Population Health and Public Health Practice, 2008.

Review of NASA's Human Research Program Evidence Books: Letter Report, Health Sciences Policy, 2008.

Review of the Use of Process Control Indicators in the FSIS Public Health Risk-Based Inspection System: Letter Report, Food and Nutrition Board, 2009.

Secondhand Smoke Exposure and Acute Coronary Events, Population Health and Public Health Practice, 2009.

The Smallpox Vaccination Program: Public Health in an Age of Terrorism, Population Health and Public Health Practice, 2005.

State of the USA Health Indicators, Letter Report, Population Health and Public Health Practice, 2008.

Toward Health Equity and Patient-Centeredness: Integrating Health Literacy, Disparities Reduction, and Quality Improvement: Workshop Summary, Population Health and Public Health Practice, 2009.

Traumatic Injury Research at NIOSH, Population Health and Public Health Practice, 2008.

Treatment of PTSD: An Assessment of the Evidence, Population Health and Public Health Practice, 2007.

Use of Dietary Supplements by Military Personnel, Food and Nutrition Board, 2008.

Vector-Borne Diseases: Understanding the Environmental, Human Health, and Ecological Connections: Workshop Summary, Global Health, 2008.

Violence Prevention in Low- and Middle-Income Countries: Finding a Place on the Global Agenda: Workshop Summary, Global Health, 2008.

Quality and patient safety

Adolescent Health Services: Missing Opportunities, Board on Children, Youth, and Families, 2008.

America's Health Care Safety Net: Intact but Endangered, Health Policy Programs and Fellowships, 2000.

America's Uninsured Crisis: Consequences for Health and Health Care, Health Care Services, 2009.

Assessing and Improving Value of Cancer Treatment: Workshop Summary, Health Care Services, 2009.

Beyond the HIPAA Privacy Rule: Enhancing Privacy, Improving Health Through Research, Health Sciences Policy, 2009.

Cancer Care for the Whole Patient: Meeting Psychosocial Health Needs, Health Care Services, 2007.

Challenges in Adolescent Health Care: Workshop Report, Board on Children, Youth, and Families, 2007.

Colorectal Cancer Screening in Average-Risk Adults: Workshop Summary, National Cancer Policy Board, IOM/NRC, 2005.

Conflict of Interest in Medical Research, Education, and Practice, Health Sciences Policy, 2009.

Creating a Business Case for Quality Improvement and Quality Improvement Research: Workshop Summary, Health Care Services, 2008.

Crossing the Quality Chasm: A New Health System for the 21st Century, Committee on Quality of Health Care in America, 2001.

The Development of DRIs 1994–2004: Lessons Learned and New Challenges: Workshop Summary, Food and Nutrition Board, 2007.

Effect of the HIPAA Privacy Rule on Health Research: Proceedings of a Workshop, National Cancer Policy Forum, 2006.

Ending the Tobacco Problem: A Blueprint for the Nation, Population Health and Public Health Practice, 2007.

Ensuring Quality Cancer Care through the Oncology Workforce: Sustaining Care in the 21st Century: Workshop Summary, National Cancer Policy Forum, 2009.

Ethical and Legal Considerations in Mitigating Pandemic Disease: Workshop Summary, Global Health, 2007.

Evidence-Based Medicine and the Changing Nature of Healthcare: Workshop Summary, Executive Office, 2008.

From Cancer Patient to Cancer Survivor: Lost in Transition, National Cancer Policy Board, 2005.

The Future of Disability in America, Health Sciences Policy, 2007.

The Future of the Public's Health in the 21st Century, Health Promotion and Disease Prevention, 2002.

Hospital-Based Emergency Care: At the Breaking Point, Health Care Services, 2007.

Improving the Social Security Disability Decision Process, Military and Veterans Health, 2007.

Insuring America's Health: Principles and Recommendations, Health Care Services, 2004.

Leadership Commitments to Improve Value in Health Care: Finding Common Ground, Workshop Summary, Evidence-Based Medicine, 2009.

Multi-Center Phase III Clinical Trials and NCI Cooperative Groups: Workshop Summary, National Cancer Policy Forum, 2009.

The National Children's Study Research Plan: A Review, Board on Children, Youth, and Families, IOM/NRC, 2008.

Opportunities for Coordination and Clarity to Advance the National Health Information Agenda: A Brief Assessment of the Office of the National Coordinator for Health Information Technology: Letter Report, Health Care Services, 2007.

Organ Donation: Opportunities for Action, Health Sciences Policy, 2006.

Preventing Childhood Obesity: Health in the Balance, Food and Nutrition Board and Board on Health Promotion and Disease Prevention, 2005.

Preventing Medication Errors: Quality Chasm Series, Health Care Services, 2006.

Preventing Teen Motor Crashes: Contributions from the Behavioral and Social Sciences, Board on Children, Youth, and Families, IOM/NRC/Transportation Research Board, 2007.

Progress in Preventing Childhood Obesity: How Do We Measure Up? Food and Nutrition Board, 2007.

Recommendations on the National Priorities for Comparative Effectiveness Research in Health Care, Health Care Services, 2009.

Redesigning the Clinical Effectiveness Research Paradigm: Innovation and Practice-Based Approaches, Executive Office, 2009.

Resident Duty Hours: Enhancing Sleep, Supervision, and Safety, Health Care Services, 2009.

Retooling for an Aging America: Building the Health Care Workforce, Health Care Services, 2008.

Reusability of Facemasks During an Influenza Pandemic: Facing the Flu, Health Sciences Policy, 2006.

A Review of the HHS Family Planning Program: Mission, Management, and Measurement of Results, Health Sciences Policy, 2009.

The Richard and Hinda Rosenthal Lecture 2008: Prospects for Health Reform in 2009 and Beyond, Executive Office, 2009.

Sleep Disorders and Sleep Deprivation: An Unmet Public Health Problem, Health Sciences Policy, 2006.

Standardized Collection of Race-Ethnicity Data for Healthcare Quality Improvement: Interim Report, Health Care Services, 2009.

Standardizing Medication Labels: Confusing Patients Less: Workshop Summary, Population Health and Public Health Practice, 2008.

The State of Quality Improvement and Implementation Research: Expert Views: Workshop Summary, Health Care Services, 2007.

State of the USA Health Indicators: Letter Report, Population Health and Public Health Practice, 2008.

Summit on Integrative Medicine and the Health of the Public: Workshop Summary, Executive Office, 2009.

To Err Is Human: Building a Safer Health System, Health Care Services, 2000.

Toward Health Equity and Patient-Centeredness: Integrating Health Literacy, Disparities Reduction, and Quality Improvement: Workshop Summary, Population Health and Public Health Practice, 2009.

Traumatic Injury Research at NIOSH, Population Health and Public Health Practice, 2008.

Use of Dietary Supplements by Military Personnel, Food and Nutrition Board, 2008.

Value in Health Care: Accounting for Cost, Quality, Safety, Outcomes, and Innovation: Workshop Summary, Evidence-Based Medicine, 2009.

Valuing Health for Regulatory Cost-Effectiveness Analysis, Health Care Services, 2006.

WIC Food Packages: Time for a Change, Food and Nutrition Board, 2005.

Select populations and health disparities

America's Health Care Safety Net: Revisiting the 2000 IOM Report, Health Care Services, 2007.

Assessment of the Role of Intermittent Preventive Treatment for Malaria in Infants: Letter Report, Global Health, 2008.

Autism and the Environment: Challenges and Opportunities for Research: Workshop Proceedings, Health Sciences Policy, 2007.

Care Without Coverage: Too Little, Too Late, Health Care Services, 2002.

Challenges and Successes in Reducing Health Disparities: Workshop Summary, Population Health and Public Health Practice, 2008.

Challenges in Adolescent Health Care: Workshop Report, Board on Children, Youth, and Families, IOM/NRC, 2007.

The Development of DRIs 1994–2004: Lessons Learned and New Challenges: Workshop Summary, Food and Nutrition Board, 2007.

Early Childhood Assessment: Why, What, and How, Board on Children, Youth, and Families, 2008.

Examining the Health Disparities Research Plan of the National Institutes of Health: Unfinished Business, Health Sciences Policy, 2006.

Foodborne Disease and Public Health: An Iranian-American Workshop, Food and Nutrition Board, 2008.

Guidance for the National Healthcare Disparities Report, Health Care Services, 2002.

Health Insurance Is a Family Matter, Health Care Services, 2002.

Investing in Children's Health: A Community Approach to Addressing Health Disparities: Workshop Summary, Population Health and Public Health Practice, 2009.

Joint U.S.-Mexico Workshop on Preventing Obesity in Children and Youth of Mexican Origin, Food and Nutrition Board, 2007.

The National Children's Study Research Plan: A Review, Board on Children, Youth, and Families, IOM/NRC, 2008.

Preterm Birth: Causes, Consequences, and Prevention, Health Sciences Policy, 2007.

Redesigning the Clinical Effectiveness Research Paradigm: Innovation and Practice-Based Approaches, Executive Office, 2009.

Retooling for an Aging America: Building the Health Care Workforce, Health Care Services, 2008.

A Review of the HHS Family Planning Program: Mission, Management, and Measurement of Results, Health Sciences Policy, 2009.

The Right Thing to Do, The Smart Thing to Do: Enhancing Diversity in Health Professions—Summary of the Symposium on Diversity in Health Professions in Honor of Herbert W. Nickens, M.D., Institute of Medicine, 2001.

Standardized Collection of Race-Ethnicity Data for Healthcare Quality Improvement: Interim Report, Health Care Services, 2009.

Standardizing Medication Labels: Confusing Patients Less: Workshop Summary, Population Health and Public Health Practice, 2008.

Toward Health Equity and Patient-Centeredness: Integrating Health Literacy, Disparities Reduction, and Quality Improvement: Workshop Summary, Population Health and Public Health Practice, 2009.

The Unequal Burden of Cancer: An Assessment of NIH Research and Programs for Ethnic Minorities and the Medically Underserved, Health Sciences Policy, 1999.

Unequal Treatment: Confronting Racial and Ethnic Disparities in Health Care, Health Sciences Policy, 2002.

Use of Dietary Supplements by Military Personnel, Food and Nutrition Board, 2008.

Substance abuse and mental health

Challenges in Adolescent Health Care: Workshop Report, Board on Children, Youth, and Families, IOM/NRC, 2007.

From Molecules to Minds: Challenges for the 21st Century: Workshop Summary, Health Sciences Policy, 2008.

From Neurons to Neighborhoods: The Science of Early Childhood Development, Board on Children, Youth, and Families, IOM/NRC, 2000.

Gulf War and Health, Volume 6: Physiologic, Psychologic, and Psychosocial Effects of Deployment-Related Stress, Population Health and Public Health Practice, 2007.

Marijuana and Medicine: Assessing the Science Base, Neuroscience and Behavioral Health, 1999.

The National Children's Study Research Plan: A Review, Board on Children, Youth, and Families, IOM/NRC, 2008.

Preventing Mental, Emotional, and Behavioral Disorders Among Young People: Progress and Possibilities, Board on Children, Youth, and Families, IOM/NRC, 2009.

Redesigning the Clinical Effectiveness Research Paradigm: Innovation and Practice-Based Approaches, Executive Office, 2009.

Treatment of PTSD: An Assessment of the Evidence, Population Health and Public Health Practice, 2007.

Use of Dietary Supplements by Military Personnel, Food and Nutrition Board, 2008.

Violence Prevention in Low- and Middle-Income Countries: Finding a Place on the Global Agenda: Workshop Summary, Global Health, 2008.

Veterans health

A 21st Century System for Evaluating Veterans for Disability Benefits, Military and Veterans Health, 2007.

Amyotrophic Lateral Sclerosis in Veterans: Review of the Scientific Literature, Population Health and Public Health Practice, 2006.

Battling Malaria: Strengthening the U.S. Military Malaria Vaccine Program, Medical Follow-Up Agency and Board on Military and Veterans Health, 2006.

Epidemiologic Studies of Veterans Exposed to Depleted Uranium: Feasibility and Design Issues, Population Health and Public Health Practice, 2008.

Gulf War and Health: Updated Literature Review of Depleted Uranium, Population Health and Public Health Practice, 2008.

Gulf War and Health, Volume 1: Depleted Uranium, Sarin, Pyridostigmine Bromide, and Vaccines, Health Promotion and Disease Prevention, 2000.

Gulf War and Health, Volume 3: Fuels, Combustion Products, and Propellants, Board on Health Promotion and Disease Prevention, 2005.

Gulf War and Health, Volume 4: Health Effects of Serving in the Gulf War, Population Health and Public Health Practice, 2006.

Gulf War and Health, Volume 5: Infectious Disease, Population Health and Public Health Practice, 2007.

🏛 **Gulf War and Health, Volume 6: Physiologic, Psychologic, and Psychosocial Effects of Deployment-Related Stress,** Population Health and Public Health Practice, 2007.

🏛 **Gulf War and Health, Volume 7: Long-term Consequences of Traumatic Brain Injury,** Population Health and Public Health Practice, 2008.

Improving the Presumptive Disability Decision-Making Process for Veterans, Military and Veterans Health, 2007.

Military Medical Ethics: Issues Regarding Dual Loyalties: Workshop Summary, Health Sciences Policy, 2008.

Posttraumatic Stress Disorder: Diagnosis and Assessment, Population Health and Public Health Practice, 2006.

PTSD Compensation and Military Service, Military and Veterans Health, 2007.

Redesigning the Clinical Effectiveness Research Paradigm: Innovation and Practice-Based Approaches, Executive Office, 2009.

Smoking Cessation in Military and Veteran Populations, Population Health and Public Health Practice, 2009.

Use of Dietary Supplements by Military Personnel, Food and Nutrition Board, 2008.

The Utility of Proximity-Based Herbicide Exposure Assessment in Epidemiologic Studies of Vietnam Veterans, Military and Veterans Health, 2008.

🏛 **Veterans and Agent Orange: Health Effects of Herbicides Used in Vietnam,** Health Promotion and Disease Prevention, 1994.

🏛 **Veterans and Agent Orange: Update 2000,** Health Promotion and Disease Prevention, 2001.

🏛 **Veterans and Agent Orange: Update 2004,** Board on Health Promotion and Disease Prevention, 2005.

🏛 **Veterans and Agent Orange: Update 2006,** Population Health and Public Health Practice, 2007.

🏛 **Veterans and Agent Orange: Update 2008,** Population Health and Public Health Practice, 2009.

Women's health

Assessing the Medical Risks of Oocyte Donation for Stem Cell Research: Workshop Report, Health Sciences Policy, 2007.

Exploring the Biological Contributions to Human Health: Does Sex Matter? Health Sciences Policy, 2001.

Improving Breast Imaging Quality Standards, National Cancer Policy Board, 2005.

Preterm Birth: Causes, Consequences, and Prevention, Health Sciences Policy, 2007.

Redesigning the Clinical Effectiveness Research Paradigm: Innovation and Practice-Based Approaches, Executive Office, 2009.

A Review of the HHS Family Planning Program: Mission, Management, and Measurement of Results, Health Sciences Policy, 2009.

Saving Women's Lives: Strategies for Improving Breast Cancer Detection and Diagnosis—A Breast Cancer Research Foundation and Institute of Medicine Symposium, National Cancer Policy Board, 2005.

Weight Gain During Pregnancy: Reexamining the Guidelines, Food and Nutrition Board, 2009.

Upcoming reports

Biomedical and health research

Cancer Clinical Trials and the NCI Cooperative Group, Health Care Services

Clinical Data as the Basic Staple of Health Learning: Creating and Protecting a Public Good: Workshop Summary, Evidence-Based Medicine

From Exposure to Human Disease: Research Strategies to Address Current Challenges, Workshop Summary, Population Health and Public Health Practice

Judging the Evidence: Standards for Determining Clinical Effectiveness: Workshop Summary, Evidence-Based Medicine

Learning What Works: Infrastructure Required to Learn Which Care Is Best: Workshop Summary, Evidence-Based Medicine

Policy Issues in the Development of Personalized Medicine in Oncology: Workshop Summary, Health Care Services

Qualification of Biomarkers as Surrogate Endpoints in Chronic Disease, Health Care Services

Review of the NIOSH Research Roadmap on Asbestos and Elongated Mineral Products, Health Sciences Policy

Children and families

Community Perspectives on Obesity Prevention in Children: Workshop Summary, Food and Nutrition Board

Nutrition Standards for National School Lunch and Breakfast Programs, Food and Nutrition Board

Diseases

Addressing the Threat of Drug Resistant Tuberculosis: Part II: Workshop Summary, Health Sciences Policy

Cancer Clinical Trials and the NCI Cooperative Group, Health Care Services

From Exposure to Human Disease: Research Strategies to Address Current Challenges: Workshop Summary, Population Health and Public Health Practice

Globalization, Movement of Pathogens (and Their Hosts) and the Revised International Health Regulations: Workshop Summary, Global Health

Policy Issues in the Development of Personalized Medicine in Oncology: Workshop Summary, Health Care Services

Preventing the Global Epidemic of Cardiovascular Disease: Meeting the Challenges in Developing Countries, Global Health

Prevention and Control of Viral Hepatitis Infections in the United States, Population Health and Public Health Practice

Public Health Priorities to Reduce and Control Hypertension, Population Health and Public Health Practice

Qualification of Biomarkers as Surrogate Endpoints in Chronic Disease, Health Care Services

Rare Diseases, Health Sciences Policy

Review of the National Vaccine Plan, Population Health and Public Health Practice

Strategies to Reduce Sodium Intake, Food and Nutrition Board

Environmental health

The Potential Impacts of Climate Change on Human Health: Workshop Summary, Population Health and Public Health Practice

Transportation Fuels and the Environment: Workshop Summary, Population Health and Public Health Practice

Food and nutrition

Community Perspectives on Obesity Prevention in Children: Workshop Summary, Food and Nutrition Board

Dietary Reference Intakes for Vitamin D and Calcium, Food and Nutrition Board

Evidence Framework for Obesity Prevention Decision Making, Food and Nutrition Board

The Food and Drug Administration's Role in Ensuring Safe Food, Food and Nutrition Board

Military Nutrition Research, Food and Nutrition Board

Mitigating the Nutritional Impacts of the Global Food Crisis: Workshop Summary, Global Health

Nutrition Standards for National School Lunch and Breakfast Programs, Food and Nutrition Board

Obesity Prevention in Texas: Workshop Summary, Food and Nutrition Board

Strategies to Reduce Sodium Intake, Food and Nutrition Board

Global health

Addressing the Threat of Drug Resistant Tuberculosis: Part II: Workshop Summary, Health Sciences Policy

Globalization, Movement of Pathogens (and Their Hosts) and the Revised International Health Regulations: Workshop Summary, Global Health

Mitigating the Nutritional Impacts of the Global Food Crisis: Workshop Summary, Global Health

Preventing the Global Epidemic of Cardiovascular Disease: Meeting the Challenges in Developing Countries, Global Health

Health care workforce

Emergency Medical Services (EMS Enterprise): Workshop Summary, Health Care Services

EMS Regionalization: Workshop Summary, Health Care Services

Future of Nursing, Executive Office

Medical Surge: Workshop Summary, Health Sciences Policy

Personal Preparedness (BARDA), Health Sciences Policy

Planning a Continuing Health Care Professional Education Institute, Health Care Services

🏛 **Qualifications or Professionals Providing Mental Health Counseling Services Under TRICARE,** Board on the Health of Select Populations

Health services, coverage, and access

Altered Standards of Care: Workshop Summary, Health Sciences Policy

Developing Trustworthy Clinical Guidelines, Health Care Services

EMS Regionalization, Workshop Summary, Health Care Services

Engineering a Learning Healthcare System: A Look at the Future: Workshop Summary, Evidence-Based Medicine

Learning What Works: Infrastructure Required to Learn Which Care Is Best: Workshop Summary, Evidence-Based Medicine

Medical Readiness, Health Sciences Policy

Medical Surge: Workshop Summary, Health Sciences Policy

Personal Preparedness (BARDA), Health Sciences Policy

Planning a Continuing Health Care Professional Education Institute, Health Care Services

Policy Issues in the Development of Personalized Medicine in Oncology: Workshop Summary, Health Care Services

Standardizing Systematic Reviews, Health Care Services

Public health

Clinical Data as the Basic Staple of Health Learning: Creating and Protecting a Public Good: Workshop Summary, Evidence-Based Medicine

Decision Making Under Uncertainty, Population Health and Public Health Practice

The Food and Drug Administration's Role in Ensuring Safe Food, Food and Nutrition Board

From Exposure to Human Disease: Research Strategies to Address Current Challenges: Workshop Summary, Population Health and Public Health Practice

Obesity Prevention in Texas: Workshop Summary, Food and Nutrition Board

The Potential Impacts of Climate Change on Human Health: Workshop Summary, Population Health and Public Health Practice

Prevention and Control of Viral Hepatitis Infections in the United States, Population Health and Public Health Practice

Public Health Priorities to Reduce and Control Hypertension, Population Health and Public Health Practice

Review of the National Vaccine Plan, Population Health and Public Health Practice

Quality and patient safety

Developing Trustworthy Clinical Guidelines, Health Care Services

Future Directions for the National Healthcare Quality and Disparities Reports, Health Care Services

Judging the Evidence: Standards for Determining Clinical Effectiveness: Workshop Summary, Evidence-Based Medicine

Learning What Works: Infrastructure Required to Learn Which Care Is Best: Workshop Summary, Evidence-Based Medicine

Qualification of Biomarkers as Surrogate Endpoints in Chronic Disease, Health Care Services

Review of the Adverse Effects of Vaccines, Population Health and Public Health Practice

Select populations and health disparities

Future Directions for the National Healthcare Quality and Disparities Reports, Health Care Services

Qualifications of Professionals Providing Mental Health Counseling Services Under TRICARE, Board on the Health of Select Populations

Substance abuse and mental health
🏛 **Qualifications of Professionals Providing Mental Health Counseling Services Under TRICARE,** Board on the Health of Select Populations

Veterans health
🏛 **Gulf War and Health: Health Effects of Serving in the Gulf War, Update 2009,** Population Health and Public Health Practice
The Initial Assessment of Readjustment Needs of Military Personnel, Veterans, and Their Families: Phase 1 and Phase 2, Population Health and Public Health Practice
Military Nutrition Research, Food and Nutrition Board

Women's health
🏛 **Women's Health Research,** Population Health and Public Health Practice

Contact Us

INSTITUTE OF MEDICINE
500 Fifth Street, N.W.
Washington, DC 20001
(202) 334-2659
www.iom.edu

Executive Office
    President: Harvey V. Fineberg, NAS-323, (202) 334-3300
    Executive Officer: Judith Salerno, NAS-325, (202) 334-2177
    Deputy Executive Officer: Clyde J. Behney, KC-838, (202) 334-2356;
    cbehney@nas.edu
    Foreign Secretary: Jo Ivey Boufford, NAS-315, (202) 334-3366
    Home Secretary: Stephen J. Ryan, NAS-316, (202) 334-2174

Office of Reports and Communications
    Director of Communications: Lauren Tobias, KC-840, (202) 334-
    2286; ltobias@nas.edu

Health Policy Educational Programs and Fellowships
    Director: Marie Michnich, KC-759, (202) 334-1296; mmichnich@
    nas.edu

Board on African Science Academy Development
    Director: Patrick Kelley, KC-850, (202) 334-2650; pkelley@nas.edu

Board on Children, Youth, and Families
    Director: Rosemary Chalk, KC-1157, (202) 334-1230; rchalk@nas.
    edu

Food and Nutrition Board
    Director: Linda Meyers, KC-740, (202) 334-3153; lmeyers@nas.edu

Board on Global Health
　　Director: Patrick Kelley, KC-850, (202) 334-2650; pkelley@nas.edu
Board on Health Care Services
　　Director: Roger Herdman, KC-758a, (202) 334-1308; rherdman@
　　nas.edu
Board on Health Sciences Policy
　　Director: Andrew Pope, KC-829, (202) 334-1739; apope@nas.edu
Board on Population Health and Public Health Practice
　　Director: Rose Marie Martinez, KC-855, (202) 334-2655; rmartinez@
　　nas.edu
Board on the Health of Select Populations
　　Director: Rick Erdtmann, KC-773, (202) 334-1925; rerdtmann@nas.
　　edu

The IOM's ability to respond quickly and independently to emerging health issues depends in part on private financial resources provided through the philanthropy of individuals, foundations, and for-profit organizations. For information on opportunities to provide philanthropic support for the IOM, please contact:

The National Academies/The Institute of Medicine Office of Development Senior Development Officer: Ellen Urbanski, KC-803, (202) 334-2371; eurbanski@nas.edu

giving@nationalacademies.org
www7.nationalacademies.org/giving